# Free access to accompanying content on www.oxfordmedicine.com/oshparkinsonsdisease2e

The copy of *Parkinson's Disease and Other Movement Disorders* you have purchased entitles you to free online access to the accompanying online video content.

Please visit:

**https://subscriberservices.sams.oup.com/token** to set up access.

To register, enter the code at the top of this card. Please keep this card for future reference as, in the event of a query, you may be asked to return it. Please note that as part of the registration process you will be informed of our terms and conditions, and will be asked to accept these to confirm your online access.

unique code: AT237элівтка

The online access provided free wit individuals who have purchased a p this will be verified as part of the a library copies should ask their libr: institution.

### Customer support

Customers outside North & Sout
**Tel:** +44 (0) 1865 353705
**Email:** accesstokens@oup.com

Customers in North & South Ar
**Tel:** 1-800-334-4249 ext. 6484
**Email:** oxfordonline@oup.com

OXFORD MEDICAL PUBLICATIONS

# Parkinson's Disease and Other Movement Disorders

# Oxford Specialist Handbooks published and forthcoming

**General Oxford Specialist Handbooks**
A Resuscitation Room Guide
Addiction Medicine
Day Case Surgery
Perioperative Medicine, 2e
Pharmaceutical Medicine
Postoperative Complications, 2e
Renal Transplantation

**Oxford Specialist Handbooks in Anaesthesia**
Anaesthesia for Medical and Surgical Emergencies
Cardiac Anaesthesia
Neuroanaesthesia
Obstetric Anaesthesia
Ophthalmic Anaesthesia
Paediatric Anaesthesia
Regional Anaesthesia, Stimulation and Ultrasound Techniques
Thoracic Anaesthesia
Vascular Anaesthesia

**Oxford Specialist Handbooks in Cardiology**
Adult Congenital Heart Disease
Cardiac Catheterization and Coronary Intervention
Cardiac Electrophysiology and Catheter Ablation
Cardiovascular Computed Tomography
Cardiovascular Magnetic Resonance
Echocardiography, 2e
Fetal Cardiology
Heart Failure
Hypertension
Inherited Cardiac Disease
Nuclear Cardiology
Pacemakers and ICDs
Pulmonary Hypertension
Valvular Heart Disease

**Oxford Specialist Handbooks in Critical Care**
Advanced Respiratory Critical Care
Cardiothoracic Critical Care

**Oxford Specialist Handbooks in End of Life Care**
End of Life Care in Cardiology
End of Life Care in Dementia
End of Life Care in Nephrology
End of Life Care in Respiratory Disease
End of Life in the Intensive Care Unit

**Oxford Specialist Handbooks in Neurology**
Epilepsy
Stroke Medicine

**Oxford Specialist Handbooks in Oncology**
Practical Management of Complex Cancer Pain

**Oxford Specialist Handbooks in Paediatrics**
Paediatric Dermatology
Paediatric Endocrinology and Diabetes
Paediatric Gastroenterology, Hepatology, and Nutrition
Paediatric Haematology and Oncology
Paediatric Intensive Care
Paediatric Nephrology, 2e
Paediatric Neurology, 2e
Paediatric Radiology
Paediatric Respiratory Medicine
Paediatric Rheumatology

**Oxford Specialist Handbooks in Pain Medicine**
Spinal Interventions in Pain Management

**Oxford Specialist Handbooks in Psychiatry**
Child and Adolescent Psychiatry
Forensic Psychiatry
Old Age Psychiatry

**Oxford Specialist Handbooks in Radiology**
Interventional Radiology
Musculoskeletal Imaging
Pulmonary Imaging
Thoracic Imaging

**Oxford Specialist Handbooks in Surgery**
Cardiothoracic Surgery, 2e
Colorectal Surgery
Gastric and Oesophageal Surgery
Hand Surgery
Hepatopancreatobiliary Surgery
Neurosurgery
Operative Surgery, 2e
Oral and Maxillofacial Surgery
Otolaryngology and Head and Neck Surgery
Paediatric Surgery
Plastic and Reconstructive Surgery
Surgical Oncology
Urological Surgery
Vascular Surgery

# Oxford Specialist Handbooks
# Parkinson's Disease and Other Movement Disorders

Second Edition

## Mark J. Edwards
Eleanor Peel Chair for the Study of Ageing, Professor of Neurology
St George's University, London, UK

## Maria Stamelou
Assistant Professor of Neurology
Philipps University, Marburg, Germany; University of Athens, Greece
Honorary Research Associate, Sobell Department of Motor Neuroscience and Movement Disorders, Institute of Neurology, University College London, UK

## Niall Quinn
Emeritus Professor of Clinical Neurology, UCL Institute of Neurology and Honorary Consultant Neurologist, National Hospital for Neurology and Neurosurgery, Queen Square, London, UK

## Kailash P. Bhatia
Professor of Clinical Neurology and Honorary Consultant Neurologist
Sobell Department of Motor Neuroscience and Movement Disorders, Institute of Neurology, University College London, UK

**OXFORD**
UNIVERSITY PRESS

# OXFORD
UNIVERSITY PRESS

Great Clarendon Street, Oxford, OX2 6DP,
United Kingdom

Oxford University Press is a department of the University of Oxford.
It furthers the University's objective of excellence in research, scholarship,
and education by publishing worldwide. Oxford is a registered trade mark of
Oxford University Press in the UK and in certain other countries

© Oxford University Press 2016

The moral rights of the authors have been asserted

First Edition published 2008
Second Edition published 2016

All rights reserved. No part of this publication may be reproduced, stored in
a retrieval system, or transmitted, in any form or by any means, without the
prior permission in writing of Oxford University Press, or as expressly permitted
by law, by licence or under terms agreed with the appropriate reprographics
rights organization. Enquiries concerning reproduction outside the scope of the
above should be sent to the Rights Department, Oxford University Press, at the
address above

You must not circulate this work in any other form
and you must impose this same condition on any acquirer

Published in the United States of America by Oxford University Press
198 Madison Avenue, New York, NY 10016, United States of America

British Library Cataloguing in Publication Data

Data available

Library of Congress Control Number: 2015945823

ISBN 978–0–19–870506–2

Printed in Great Britain by
Ashford Colour Press Ltd, Gosport, Hampshire

Oxford University Press makes no representation, express or implied, that the
drug dosages in this book are correct. Readers must therefore always check
the product information and clinical procedures with the most up-to-date
published product information and data sheets provided by the manufacturers
and the most recent codes of conduct and safety regulations. The authors and
the publishers do not accept responsibility or legal liability for any errors in the
text or for the misuse or misapplication of material in this work. Except where
otherwise stated, drug dosages and recommendations are for the non-pregnant
adult who is not breast-feeding

Links to third party websites are provided by Oxford in good faith and
for information only. Oxford disclaims any responsibility for the materials
contained in any third party website referenced in this work.

# Preface and acknowledgements

In some ways, movement disorders are amongst the most obvious of neurological disorders; without any special examination techniques above those of simple observation, most movement disorders can be readily appreciated. But what then? How can one take these basic observations and translate them into diagnostic formulations, appropriate investigation, and even treatment? In a specialty where there are few diagnostic tests, and where lists of differential diagnoses of the six main movement disorders seem to expand every week, how does the clinician approach the patient with a movement disorder?

This book is designed to guide the reader through this process. Throughout the book, we have attempted to build a route from careful targeted history taking and examination through to appropriate investigation and practical treatment advice. As an aid to this, we have provided online videos of patients with different movement disorders. Although we have kept a focus on the commoner movement disorders, in particular Parkinson's disease, we have also made sure that the book is comprehensive by including details of rarer movement disorders, highlighting their clinical features and explaining when they should be considered in the differential diagnosis.

This 'approach to movement disorders' is the way in which we teach our own students and clinical fellows in the clinic. It has developed from our own experience, but also from that of our teachers. In this regard, we wish to acknowledge the great debt that we all owe to Professor David Marsden, who did so much to advance the clinical and pathophysiological knowledge of movement disorders.

We also wish to acknowledge our gratitude to our patients, particularly those who agreed for their videos to be included in this book, those consultants who kindly provided videos, including Steve Tisch and Ying-Zu Huang, Dr Penelope Talelli for her assistance with the preparation of the figures and videos, and to Pete Stevenson, Lauren Dunn, and Rachel Goldsworthy at Oxford University Press for their dedication and efficiency in guiding this book to its completion.

MJJE
MS
NPQ
KPB

# Authors' disclaimer*

Note that, within this book, off-licence use of drugs is described, and dosages of some medications are in excess of typically recommended doses. This reflects clinical practice, but practitioners should always consult local and national prescription guidelines and seek pharmaceutical advice before off-licence prescription or prescription of higher than typically recommended doses of medication.

* Whenever an asterisk is denoted in the text, please refer back to this authors' disclaimer.

# Dedication

To our families—present and future.

MJJE
MS
NPQ
KPB

# Contents

Symbols and abbreviations x

| | | |
|---|---|---|
| 1 | Approach to patients with movement disorders | 1 |
| 2 | Anatomy and function of the basal ganglia | 9 |
| 3 | Parkinson's disease | 21 |
| 4 | Atypical parkinsonism | 93 |
| 5 | Tremor | 123 |
| 6 | Tics | 141 |
| 7 | Chorea | 159 |
| 8 | Myoclonus | 175 |
| 9 | Dystonia | 195 |
| 10 | Drug-induced movement disorders | 249 |
| 11 | Paroxysmal movement disorders | 267 |
| 12 | Movement disorders and ataxia | 279 |
| 13 | Movement disorders and sleep | 291 |
| 14 | Other dyskinetic syndromes | 303 |
| 15 | Functional (psychogenic) movement disorders | 313 |
| 16 | Startle and stiff-person syndromes | 329 |

Index 335

# Symbols and abbreviations

| | |
|---|---|
| * | Please refer to the authors' disclaimer on page vi |
| ABGA | anti-basal ganglia antibody |
| AC | akinetic crisis |
| ADHD | attention-deficit/hyperactivity disorder |
| ADNFLE | autosomal dominant nocturnal frontal lobe epilepsy |
| ADR | acute dystonic reaction |
| AHC | alternating hemiplegia of childhood |
| ALS | amyotrophic lateral sclerosis |
| AMRF | action myoclonus renal failure syndrome |
| AOA | ataxia with oculomotor apraxia |
| APS | antiphospholipid syndrome |
| ASO | anti-streptolysin O |
| AT | ataxia telangiectasia |
| bd | twice daily |
| *BNF* | *British National Formulary* |
| BP | *bereitschafts* potential |
| BPAN | beta-propeller protein-associated neurodegeneration |
| BT | botulinum toxin |
| CBD | corticobasal degeneration |
| CBS | corticobasal syndrome |
| CDS | continuous dopaminergic stimulation |
| CIDP | chronic inflammatory demyelinating polyradiculoneuropathy |
| CJD | Creutzfeldt–Jakob disease |
| CK | creatine kinase |
| cm | centimetre |
| CNS | central nervous system |
| COMT | catechol-*O*-methyltransferase |
| CSF | cerebrospinal fluid |
| CSM | Committee on Safety of Medicines |
| CT | computerized tomography |
| DAT | dopamine transporter protein |

| | |
|---|---|
| DBS | deep brain stimulation |
| DLB | dementia with Lewy bodies |
| DNA | deoxyribonucleic acid |
| DRB | dopamine receptor-blocking drug |
| DRD | dopa-responsive dystonia |
| DRPLA | dentatorubropallidoluysian atrophy |
| *DSM* | *Diagnostic and Statistical Manual of Mental Disorders* |
| DWI | diffusion-weighted imaging |
| EA1 | episodic ataxia type 1 |
| EA2 | episodic ataxia type 2 |
| EA5 | episodic ataxia type 5 |
| ECG | electrocardiography |
| EEG | electroencephalography |
| EMG | electromyography |
| EPC | epilepsia partialis continua |
| ESR | erythrocyte sedimentation rate |
| ET | essential tremor |
| FDFM | familial dyskinesia facial myokymia |
| FDG | 18-fluorodeoxyglucose |
| FHM1 | familial hemiplegic migraine 1 |
| FMD | functional movement disorder |
| FTD | fronto-temporal dementia |
| FTDP-17 | fronto-temporal dementia linked to chromosome 17q |
| FUS | fused-in sarcoma |
| FXTAS | fragile X-associated tremor/ataxia syndrome |
| g | gram |
| GABA | gamma-aminobutyric acid |
| GAD | glutamic acid decarboxylase |
| GBA | glucocerebrosidase |
| GP | general practitioner |
| GLUT1 | glucose transporter 1 |
| GPe | external segment of the globus pallidus |
| GPi | internal segment of the globus pallidus |
| HARP | hypoprebetalipoproteinaemia, acanthocytosis, retinitis pigmentosa, pallidal degeneration |
| HD | Huntington's disease |

| | |
|---|---|
| HDU | high-dependency unit |
| 5-HIAA | 5-hydroxyindoleacetic acid |
| HIV | human immunodeficiency virus |
| HPRT | hypoxanthine–guanine phosphoribosyltransferase |
| HSMN | hereditary sensorimotor neuropathy |
| HSP | hereditary spastic paraplegia |
| HVA | homovanillic acid |
| Hz | hertz (cycle per second) |
| IBGC | idiopathic basal ganglia calcification |
| IBZM | iodobenzamide |
| ICD | impulse control disorder |
| ICU | intensive care unit |
| IF | intermediate filament |
| IgM | immunoglobulin M |
| INAD | infantile neuroaxonal dystrophy |
| IV | intravenous |
| IVIG | intravenous immunoglobulin |
| kg | kilogram |
| LDL | low-density lipoprotein |
| LSVT | Lee Silverman Voice Treatment |
| m | metre |
| MAG | myelin-associated glycoprotein |
| MAO | monoamine oxidase |
| MAO-A | monoamine oxidase A |
| MAO-B | monoamine oxidase B |
| MAOI | monoamine oxidase inhibitor |
| MAPT | microtubule-associated protein tau |
| MERRF | myoclonus epilepsy with ragged red fibres |
| mg | milligram |
| MIBG | [123]meta-iodobenzylguanidine |
| mL | millilitre |
| mmHg | millimetre of mercury |
| MPAN | mitochondrial membrane protein-associated neurodegeneration |
| MPTP | 1-methyl-4-phenyl-1,2,3,6-tetrahydropyridine |
| MRI | magnetic resonance imaging |

| | |
|---|---|
| ms | millisecond |
| MSA | multiple system atrophy |
| MU | mega unit |
| NBIA | neuronal brain iron accumulation syndrome |
| NCL | neuronal ceroid lipofuscinosis |
| NHS | National Health Service |
| NICE | National Institute for Health and Care Excellence |
| NIFID | neuronal intermediate filament inclusion disease |
| NIID | neuronal intranuclear inclusion disease |
| NMDA | *N*-methyl-*D*-aspartic acid |
| NMS | neuroleptic malignant syndrome |
| NOSI | non-obscene, socially inappropriate behaviours |
| OCD | obsessive–compulsive disorder |
| OMM | oculo-masticatory myorhythmia |
| OT | orthostatic tremor |
| PAGF | pure akinesia with gait freezing |
| PANDAS | paediatric autoimmune neuropsychiatric disorder associated with streptococcal infection |
| PAPT | progressive ataxia palatal tremor syndrome |
| PD | Parkinson's disease |
| PDD | Parkinson's disease-associated dementia |
| PIGD | postural instability and gait disturbance |
| PD-MCI | Parkinson's disease with mild cognitive impairment |
| PDNS | Parkinson's disease nurse specialist |
| PED | paroxysmal exercise-induced dyskinesia |
| PEG | percutaneous endoscopic gastroscopy |
| PERM | progressive encephalomyelitis with rigidity and myoclonus |
| PET | positron emission tomography |
| PHS | parkinsonism–hyperpyrexia syndrome |
| PKAN | panthonate kinase-associated neurodegeneration |
| PKD | paroxysmal kinesigenic dyskinesia |
| PLAN | phospholipase 2, group VI-associated neurodegeneration |
| PLMS | periodic limb movements of sleep |
| PMEA | progressive myoclonic epilepsy–ataxia syndrome |

| | |
|---|---|
| PNFA | progressive non-fluent aphasia |
| PNKD | paroxysmal non-kinesigenic dyskinesia |
| PPN | pedunculopontine nucleus |
| PSP | progressive supranuclear palsy |
| RBD | REM-sleep behaviour disorder |
| REM | rapid eye movement |
| RLS | restless legs syndrome |
| RODP | rapid-onset dystonia parkinsonism |
| RS | Richardson's syndrome |
| SCA | spinocerebellar ataxia |
| SDS | Shy–Drager syndrome |
| SLE | systemic lupus erythematosus |
| SLT | speech and language therapy |
| SNc | substantia nigra pars compacta |
| SNr | substantia nigra pars reticulata |
| SNRI | serotonin and noradrenaline reuptake inhibitor |
| sOPCA | sporadic olivopontocerebellar atrophy |
| SPECT | single-photon emission computerized tomography |
| SPS | stiff-person syndrome |
| SRD | sepiapterin reductase deficiency |
| SS | serotonin syndrome |
| SSEP | somatosensory evoked potential |
| SSPE | subacute sclerosing panencephalitis |
| SSRI | selective serotonin reuptake inhibitor |
| STN | subthalamic nucleus |
| SWEDD | scan without evidence of dopaminergic deficit |
| T | tesla |
| tds | three times daily |
| TENS | transcutaneous electrical nerve stimulation |
| THB | tetrahydrobiopterin |
| TS | Tourette's syndrome |
| UK | United Kingdom |
| UPDRS | Unified Parkinson's Disease Rating Scale |
| VIM | ventro-intermediate nucleus |
| WD | Wilson's disease |

# Digital media accompanying the book

Individual purchasers of this book are entitled to free personal access to accompanying digital media in the online edition. Please refer to the access token card for instructions on token redemption and access.

These online ancillary materials, where available, are noted with iconography throughout the book.

- Video

The corresponding media can be found on *Oxford Medicine Online* at: http://www.oxfordmedicine.com/oshparkinsonsdisease2e.

If you are interested in access to the complete online edition, please consult with your librarian.

# Chapter 1

# Approach to patients with movement disorders

Which movement disorder is it? 2
Approach to the investigation of movement disorders 4
Approach to the management of movement disorders 6

# Which movement disorder is it?

## Step 1: Hypokinetic versus hyperkinetic movement disorders

The simplest way to categorize patients with movement disorders is into those with too little movement, *hypokinetic*, or those with too much movement, *hyperkinetic*. The hyperkinetic movement disorders as a group are often called *dyskinesias*.

## Step 2: Which type of hypo-/hyperkinetic movement disorder?

Six main movement disorders are recognized.

### Hypokinetic
- **Parkinsonism**, also called **akinetic–rigid syndrome**. A syndrome comprising akinesia (slowness, fatiguing, and decrement of repetitive movements) as an obligatory feature, also rigidity, and often, in addition, tremor and gait disturbance.

### Hyperkinetic
- **Tremor**: rhythmic sinusoidal oscillation of a body part.
- **Tics**: involuntary stereotyped movements or vocalizations.
- **Chorea**: brief irregular, purposeless movements which flit and flow from one body part to another.
- **Myoclonus**: brief electric shock-like jerks.
- **Dystonia**: abnormal posture of the affected body part.

## Pitfalls
- Some movement disorders can look very similar. For example, it can be difficult to distinguish among jerks (tics, chorea, and myoclonus), or between rhythmic myoclonus and tremor. Throughout the book, guidance is given on clinical methods to distinguish between different movement disorders. The online videos that accompany this book will also aid recognition of the clinical features of each of the movement disorders.
- Some patients have 'mixed movement disorders'. For example, tics and chorea may occur together in patients with neuroacanthocytosis. In such cases, it is often useful to ask the question 'What is the main movement disorder present?', and to consider the patient in light of this main disorder.

## Step 3: Forming a differential diagnosis

A quick look at any of the chapters in this book dealing with the major movement disorders will reveal a long list of possible causes for each disorder. The role of careful history taking and examination is to help reduce this list to a few likely diagnoses, and each chapter contains a guide to history taking and examination for each movement disorder which will help you perform this important task.

When attempting to form a list of possible causes of a movement disorder in a particular patient, it is helpful to remember that, in general, causes of movement disorders fall into four categories:

- **Primary (idiopathic)**: these tend to be 'pure' movement disorders (no other neurological/systemic features such as cognitive decline, epilepsy, spasticity, organ failure) that are non-progressive and usually do not have structural brain lesions. These disorders are often inherited. The term primary replaced the older term idiopathic. However, there is a trend to also abandon the term primary and instead use the term isolated, to highlight the absence of other signs, without making assumptions about the underlying aetiology.
- **Secondary**: these are movement disorders caused by identifiable secondary causes such as brain injury, infection, or drug use. Other systems may be involved, and other neurological signs may occur. The defining feature of these conditions is the presence of a precipitating factor, although remember that movement disorders can have a delayed onset after the precipitating event. Secondary movement disorders are usually static and do not progress if the precipitating factor is no longer active.
- **Heredo-degenerative**: these are movement disorders which occur as part of a generalized degenerative process affecting the nervous system. Clinical presentation is often very variable in these disorders, and the movement disorder may only be a minor part of the neurological/systemic dysfunction. These disorders cause progressive disability.
- **Psychogenic**: an important cause of movement disorders which has a diverse presentation, usually coupled with other unusual physical symptoms and signs, and sometimes the additional presence of psychological disturbance.

# Approach to the investigation of movement disorders

There are two incorrect, but commonly practised, and opposite approaches to the investigation of movement disorders:
- Exhaustively going down the list of possible tests to make sure that no possible diagnosis is missed, however distant the patient's phenotype is from the recognized phenotype of the disorder being tested for
- Considering that most patients with a movement disorder will have the common cause for this (e.g. most patients with parkinsonism will have Parkinson's disease (PD), most patients with tremor will have essential tremor (ET)), and therefore no investigation is necessary.

Both these approaches can ultimately fail the patient. It is self-evident that most patients with a particular movement disorder will have a common cause for it. It is therefore of great importance for the practitioner to have a thorough knowledge of the clinical spectrum of common movement disorders. With this, the practitioner will be able to diagnose such patients with confidence *and* identify that small group of patients who do not fit the typical pattern of the common disorder and require further investigation.

## Planning investigations
- **Could there be a treatable cause for the movement disorder?** There are few treatable movement disorders (e.g. PD, Wilson's disease (WD), dopa-responsive dystonia (DRD)); therefore, there should be a high index of suspicion for these, and they should be a priority for appropriate investigation.
- **Consider syndromic associations.** The differential diagnosis of heredo-degenerative movement disorders is usually very long, and investigating all the possibilities would be expensive, and hugely time-consuming and unpleasant for the patient. In such cases, it is very helpful to consider whether the patient has other symptoms or signs that can help to narrow the differential diagnosis. For example, the differential diagnosis of a patient with heredo-degenerative dystonia *and* peripheral neuropathy is much shorter than that of heredo-degenerative dystonia in general.
- **Manage the patient's expectations.** Patients may happily undergo heroic investigation with large numbers of expensive and invasive tests, as they expect that finding the diagnosis will enable effective treatment. Unfortunately, this is often not the case. Many patients wish to have a 'label' for their condition, and investigation to try to achieve this is reasonable. However, at each stage of the investigation process, expectations should be managed, and the option of a temporary or permanent halt to the investigations should be discussed.

# Approach to the management of movement disorders

The majority of movement disorders are amenable to symptomatic treatment only. Few are curable, and, in many, progression of symptoms occurs over time. In view of this, an honest partnership between patient and physician is needed which accepts the limitations of treatment and explores the full range of options available. This range of options includes no treatment or withdrawal of treatment.

## Supportive treatment
- Deciding not to take treatment is a reasonable option for many patients. Patients may be concerned that not taking treatment will affect the course of the underlying condition. This is almost always not the case, and patients should be reassured in this regard.
- Many patients find that patient support associations are very helpful, and information regarding the 'official' organizations is given at the end of each chapter. Patients should be warned about the dangers of poor-quality information on the Internet and from other sources, and to treat claims of expensive miracle cures and treatments with caution.
- Patients with movement disorders may need assistance from social services and may be entitled to disability benefits. Such services often require a diagnosis and prognosis to be given, before help becomes available. Given the difficulty in a precise diagnosis in movement disorders, a general description of the condition, e.g. 'progresssive generalized dystonia', can serve as a diagnosis and can be a great help to patients in achieving an adequate level of social and financial support.

## Medical treatment
- For most movement disorders, apart from PD, a small range of symptomatic treatments are available.
- The key to a successful trial of medication is to start with a small dose and build up slowly.
- Starting with too high a dose or building up too quickly will usually lead to unpleasant side effects, and often the patient will be unwilling to take the medication again, even at a lower dose. With so few treatment options, one cannot afford to miss out on a proper trial of a particular medication because of lack of care in dose selection and titration.
- Slow titration should continue, until sufficient benefit occurs or unacceptable side effects arise. If side effects occur with no benefit to symptoms, the medication can be withdrawn, and a trial of another medication attempted if the patient wishes.
- It is important that patients understand the 'trial and error' approach to symptomatic treatment of movement disorders. If this is not explained, patients may have unreasonably high expectations of benefit. If the medication fails to deliver, the patient can lose trust in the clinician and be unwilling to try further treatment.

## Botulinum toxin treatment
- Botulinum toxin (BT) has been a remarkable advance in the treatment of those with focal dystonia (especially if it affects muscles of the face or neck). It has a much more limited application for other forms of dystonia and for other movement disorders.

## Surgical treatment
- Lesion operations of the basal ganglia can be effective for some movement disorders (in particular, PD, dystonia, and tremor), but such operations can cause significant serious side effects (e.g. brain injury).
- Lesion operations have now been largely replaced by deep brain stimulation (DBS) where electrodes are inserted into the basal ganglia and connected to implanted electrical pulse generators.
- DBS causes intraoperative brain damage and haemorrhage much less commonly, compared with lesion operations. Hardware complications, such as lead infection and fracture, may occur. DBS is an expensive procedure and is not universally available.
- Correct selection of patients for DBS is essential to ensure the maximum chance of success, but, if this is done, the procedure does offer significant and lasting benefits for some carefully selected patients with particular movement disorders.

# Chapter 2

# Anatomy and function of the basal ganglia

Structure and function of the basal ganglia *10*
Basal ganglia circuits *14*
Basal ganglia circuits and movement disorders *18*
Neurotransmitters in the basal ganglia *20*

# Structure and function of the basal ganglia

### Where are the basal ganglia?
The basal ganglia are a group of interconnected structures which occupy an area between the cortex and brainstem in the centre of the brain (Fig. 2.1).

### What structures make up the basal ganglia?
Fig. 2.2 shows the position of the various structures that make up the basal ganglia. These are as follows:

- Caudate nucleus
- Putamen
- Globus pallidus interna and externa
- Subthalamic nucleus (STN)
- Substantia nigra pars compacta (SNc) and pars reticulata (SNr)
- Ventrolateral nucleus of the thalamus.

The caudate and putamen are together called the *striatum*. The putamen and globus pallidus are together called the *lentiform nucleus*.

### What do the basal ganglia do?
- The basal ganglia receive a huge number of inputs, mainly from the cortex, and produce a much smaller number of outputs, mainly back to the cortex, but also directly to the brainstem and the cerebellum.
- The basal ganglia are therefore part of an 'information loop', taking information from the cortex, processing it, and then passing information back.
- One major role of the basal ganglia appears to be in mediating automatic activity (habitual control). For example, learning to drive a car is initially an entirely conscious voluntary activity (goal-directed), but, with time, it becomes a largely automatic process.
- The basal ganglia are involved in much more than just movement. This explains the cognitive and psychiatric problems commonly experienced by those with movement disorders.
- There are a number of basal ganglia loops, taking information from different parts of the cortex and feeding it back again:
  - **motor loop**: control of movement
  - **oculomotor loop**: component of eye movement control
  - **lateral orbito-frontal loop**: control of social behaviour, implicated in obsessive–compulsive disorder (OCD)
  - **dorsolateral prefrontal loop**: control of executive function, planning, working memory
  - **anterior cingulate loop**: role unclear—may help to reinforce signals from other basal ganglia loops, especially the motor loop.

- An important aspect of the functional organization of these loops is their spatial topography which is maintained throughout the loop. Cortical regions associated with sensorimotor, limbic (emotional), and associative (cognitive) functions provide topographically ordered input to the posterior putamen, ventral striatum, and caudate and anterior putamen, respectively (Fig. 2.3).
- The basal ganglia also receive input from the brainstem (superior and inferior colliculi, periaqueductal grey, pedunculopontine nucleus, locus coeruleus, pontine and medullary reticular nuclei) and the thalamus.

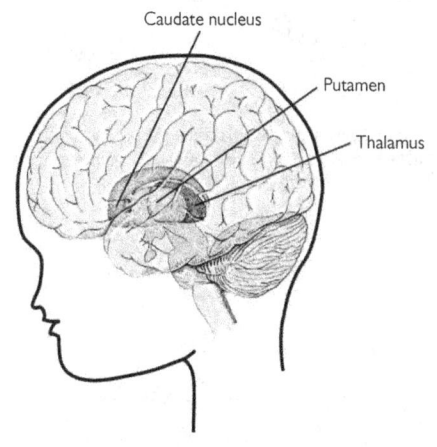

**Fig. 2.1** Position of the basal ganglia within the brain.

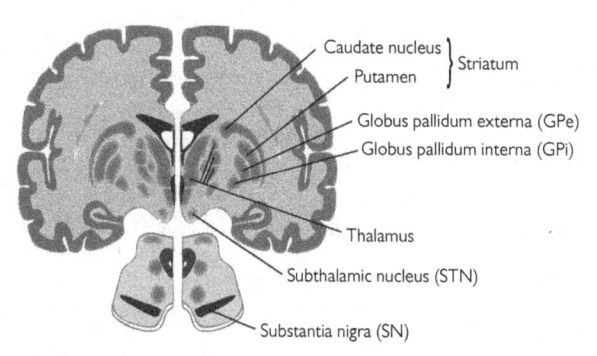

**Fig. 2.2** Components of the basal ganglia seen in a coronal section of the brain.

## CHAPTER 2 **Anatomy & function of the basal ganglia**

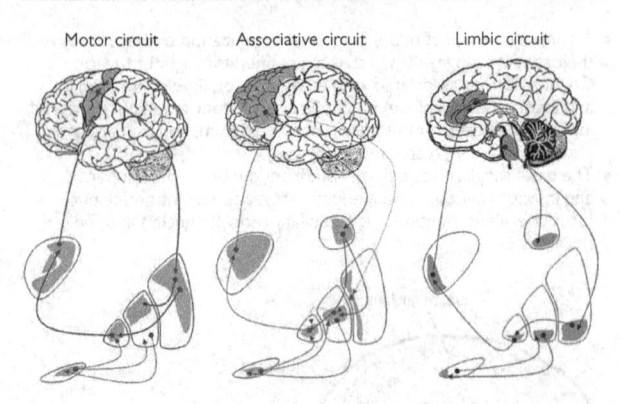

**Fig. 2.3** Spatial organization of the basal ganglia and cortex.

Adapted from *The Lancet*, **384**(9942) Obeso JA et al., The expanding universe of disorders of the basal ganglia, pp. 523–531, Copyright (2014), with permission from Elsevier.

# Basal ganglia circuits

There are complex connections between the various components of the basal ganglia: the basal ganglia circuits. The precise function of these circuits and how dysfunction causes movement disorders are the subject of intense ongoing debate. However, models of basal ganglia circuits have been produced which help to explain, albeit imperfectly, how damage to particular parts of the basal ganglia can cause movement disorders.

### Input and output

One of the simplest ways to think about basal ganglia circuits is to consider that they have structures which act as inputs (information from the cortex enters the system here) and outputs (information processed by the basal ganglia exits from here). The **caudate** and **putamen** (together called the **striatum**) are the main input structures. The **internal segment of the globus pallidus (GPi)** is the main output structure.

### Internal segment of the globus pallidus is an inhibitory structure

It is essential to understand that the GPi is an inhibitory structure. It projects to, and inhibits, the thalamus, which connects through excitatory neurons to the cortex. Therefore, an *increase* in activity in the GPi will cause a *decrease* in thalamic and cortical activity, and a *decrease* in activity in the GPi will cause an *increase* in thalamic and cortical activity.

### Direct and indirect pathways

There are two major pathways between the input structures (striatum) and output structures (GPi):
- **the direct pathway**: this is a direct link between the striatum and the GPi. Activity in this pathway *inhibits* the Gpi (Fig. 2.4)
- **the indirect pathway**: this is an indirect link between the striatum and the GPi, going via the external segment of the globus pallidus (GPe) and the STN. The net result of activity in this pathway is to *excite* the GPi (Fig. 2.4).

*Direct and indirect pathways have opposite effects on the cortex*
The direct pathway can be thought of as the 'go' pathway, as activity here will decrease GPi activity, therefore increasing thalamic and cortical activity and promoting movement. The indirect pathway is the 'stop' pathway, as activity here increases GPi activity, reducing thalamic and cortical activity, and therefore reducing movement.

*Dopamine has opposite effects on the direct and indirect pathways*
Dopaminergic neurons project from the SNc to the striatum. Here, they synapse with neurons from the direct and indirect pathways (Fig. 2.5).
- The direct pathway has D1 dopamine receptors. When dopamine binds to these, *the direct pathway is activated*.
- The indirect pathway has D2 dopamine receptors. When dopamine binds to these, *the indirect pathway is inhibited*.
- Therefore, the overall effect of dopamine is to *decrease* GPi activity, thereby *promoting* movement.

### New knowledge on basal ganglia circuits

- Although the direct and indirect pathways remain valid, it is now recognized that they represent only a subset of connections between the basal ganglia nuclei, albeit an important one.
- The basal ganglia can no longer be seen as an exclusively feed-forward structure with unidirectional connections along the cortico–basal ganglia–thalamo–cortical circuit, since there is now clear evidence of reciprocal connections between the nuclei.
  - An important additional feature of the direct pathway from the striatum to the output nuclei (GPi and SNr) are collateral fibres to the GPe (Fig. 2.6).
  - The STN is no longer considered just a station between the GPe and the GPi in the indirect pathway but is recognized as a major input structure, receiving input directly from the cortex (hyperdirect pathway), thalamus, and brainstem structures (Fig. 2.6).
  - The GPe projects not only to the STN, but also directly to the GPi, and SNr, and to nigrostriatal dopamine neurons (Fig. 2.6).

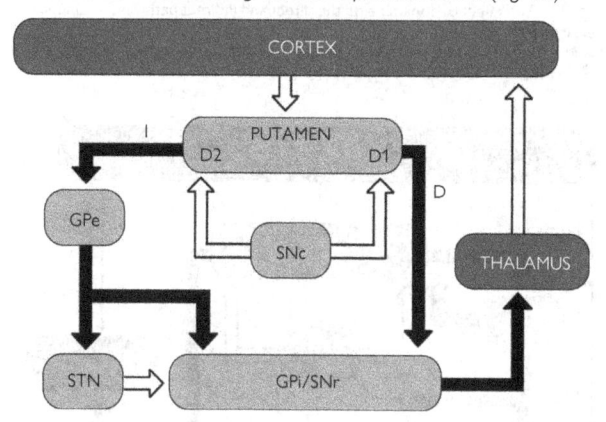

**Fig. 2.4** The direct and indirect pathways. Black arrows indicate inhibitory connections, and white arrows indicate excitatory connections. D, direct pathway; I, indirect pathway; D1, dopamine receptor type 1; D2, dopamine receptor type 2; GPe, globus pallidus externa; GPi, globus pallidus interna; SNc, substantia nigra pars compacta; SNr, substantia nigra pars reticulata; STN, subthalamic nucleus.

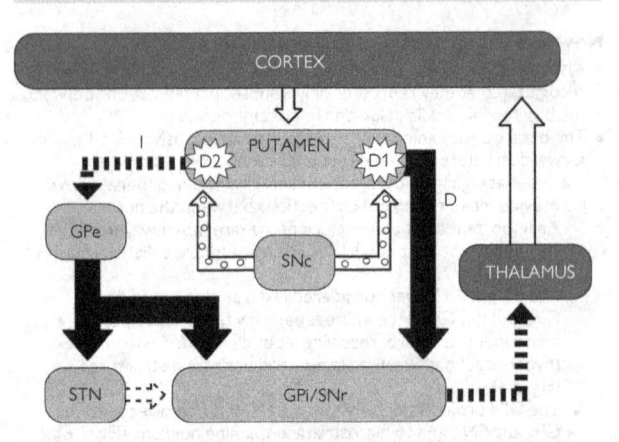

**Fig. 2.5** The effect of dopamine on the direct and indirect pathways. Dopamine released from the substantia nigra pars compacta stimulates the direct pathway via its action on D1 receptors, and inhibits the indirect pathway via its action on D2 receptors. Abbreviations are as in Fig. 2.4.

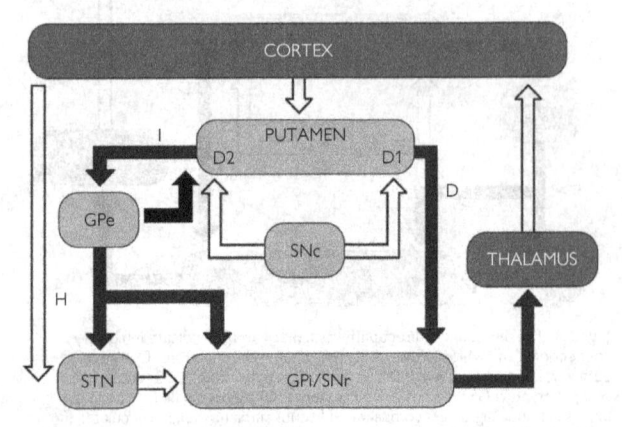

**Fig. 2.6** The reciprocal connections between the basal ganglia, beyond the direct and indirect pathways. H, hyperdirect pathway.

# Basal ganglia circuits and movement disorders

### Hypokinetic movement disorders
Dopamine has different effects on the direct and indirect pathways, and tends to promote movement by reducing GPi activity. In PD (see Video 2.1: Parkinson's disease), the SNc is damaged, and this reduces dopaminergic stimulation of the striatum (Fig. 2.7). As a result, direct ('go') pathway activity is reduced, and indirect ('stop') pathway activity is increased. This leads to an increase in GPi activity, and therefore inhibition of the thalamus and cortex. This is hypothesized to lead to the slowness of movement seen in PD.

### Hyperkinetic movement disorders
Hemiballismus is a hyperkinetic movement disorder characterized by wild flinging movements of the limbs (see Video 2.1: Parkinson's disease). A lesion of the STN is often seen in these patients. Fig. 2.8 shows how this lesion might cause excessive movement. Destruction of the STN will reduce indirect ('stop') pathway activity, leaving the direct ('go') pathway unopposed. This will reduce GPi output, thereby increasing thalamic and cortical activity, and promoting movement.

### Problems with basal ganglia models
The simple model of basal ganglia circuits presented has a number of difficulties. For example:
- a surgical lesion of GPi can improve a hyperkinetic movement disorder, such as dystonia, as well as a hypokinetic movement disorder such as PD
- the model cannot explain the variety of hyperkinetic disorders. Why do some patients with basal ganglia dysfunction develop tremor, while others develop chorea?

### Emerging concepts
- These inconsistencies have led to the idea that the pathophysiology of movement disorders may not be solely explained by changes in the firing rate of the STN/GPi, but they may also involve abnormal oscillatory patterns of neuronal activity.
- Specific interest exists for beta oscillations. Their physiological role is proposed to be the maintenance of the current motor state or 'status quo'. Elevated beta is associated with slowing of spontaneous movements.
- Phasic release of dopamine is associated with beta suppression and promotion of change in the movement state (e.g. initiating a new movement, changing from one movement pattern to another).
- Recordings from DBS macro-electrodes in PD patients have shown increased beta activity in patients withdrawn from dopaminergic medication, and a suppression of beta activity by levodopa and DBS in proportion to clinical improvement.
- Thus, the emerging hypothesis in movement disorders is that these may reflect abnormalities in synchronized oscillatory activity.

BASAL GANGLIA CIRCUITS AND MOVEMENT DISORDERS 19

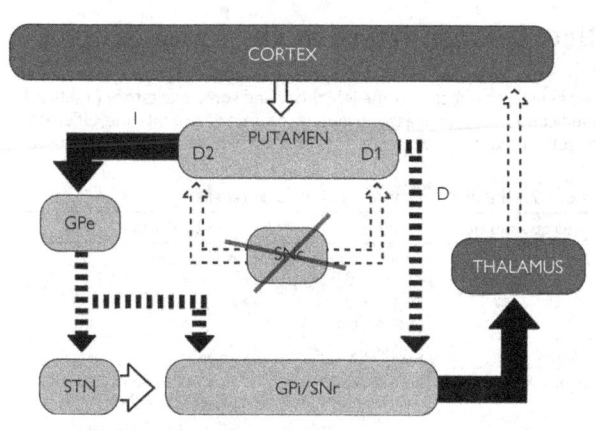

**Fig. 2.7** How a lesion in the substantia nigra pars compacta can cause parkinsonism. Abbreviations are as in Fig. 2.4.

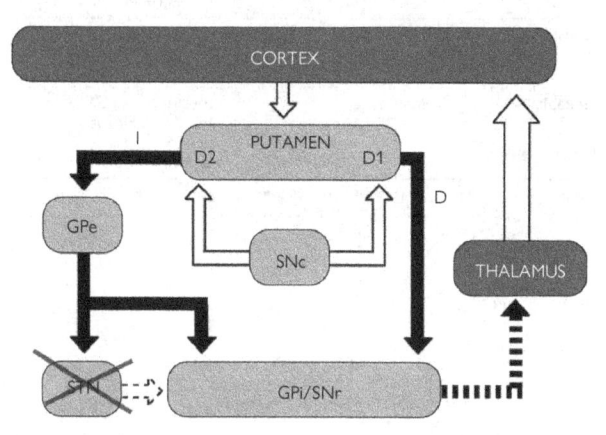

**Fig. 2.8** How a lesion in the subthalamic nucleus can cause hemiballismus. Abbreviations are as in Fig. 2.4.

# Neurotransmitters in the basal ganglia

Neurons connecting the various structures of the basal ganglia use different neurotransmitters, some inhibitory and some excitatory (Table 2.1). Medication used to treat movement disorders exploits the differential effects of these neurotransmitters on the function of the basal ganglia.

Table 2.1 Neurotransmitters in the basal ganglia

| Neurotransmitter | Action | Site of action |
| --- | --- | --- |
| Dopamine | Excitatory to D1 receptors (direct pathway) | Striatum |
| | Inhibitory to D2 receptors (indirect pathway) | |
| Acetylcholine | Excitatory | Striatum |
| GABA | Inhibitory | Links striatum with GPi (direct pathway) |
| | | Links striatum with GPe, GPe, and STN (indirect pathway), and with GPi and thalamus |
| Substance P | Inhibitory | Localized with GABA in neurons linking striatum and GPi (direct pathway) |
| Enkephalin | Inhibitory | Localized with GABA in neurons linking striatum and GPe (indirect pathway) |

GABA, gamma-aminobutyric acid; GPe, external segment of globus pallidus; GPi, internal segment of globus pallidus; STN, subthalamic nucleus.

## Chapter 3

# Parkinson's disease

Introduction 22
Approach to the patient with parkinsonism 24
Parkinson's disease 26
Pathophysiology of Parkinson's disease 28
Parkinson's disease: history 30
Parkinson's disease: examination 32
Parkinson's disease: clinical diagnosis 34
Non-motor symptoms in Parkinson's disease: dementia 36
Other non-motor symptoms in Parkinson's disease 38
Parkinson's disease: investigations 40
Genetics of Parkinson's disease 42
Breaking the news 46
Management of Parkinson's disease 48
Treatment of motor symptoms 50
Levodopa 52
Dopamine agonists: 1 56
Dopamine agonists: 2 58
Monoamine oxidase inhibitors 60
Catechol-O-methyltransferase inhibitors 62
Amantadine and the anticholinergics 64
Treatment initiation 66
Treatment of non-motor symptoms 68
Physiotherapy, occupational therapy, and speech therapy 70
Follow-up of patients with Parkinson's disease 72
Treatment escalation 74
Management of dyskinesias 78
Non-motor side effects of dopaminergic therapy 80
Apomorphine 82
Duodopa® 84
Deep brain stimulation 86
The Parkinson's disease nurse specialist 88
Measuring Parkinson's disease severity 90
Useful websites and addresses 92

# CHAPTER 3 **Parkinson's disease**

# Introduction

## What is parkinsonism?

The fundamental feature of parkinsonism is **akinesia**.

- **Akinesia**: this term includes *bradykinesia* (slowness of movement), poverty of movement, and, most importantly, *fatiguing and decrement in size of repetitive movement*. It is usually demonstrated clinically by asking the patient to perform a rapid alternating movement such as repetitively opposing index finger and thumb. Simple slowness of movement can occur in other conditions (e.g. spasticity). It is the progressive decrease in the amplitude and fatiguing of speed of movement that is essential to diagnose akinesia.

There are three other components of parkinsonism that may or may not be present.

- **Rigidity**: this is a feeling of resistance when moving the patient's relaxed limb. The rigidity in parkinsonism is often described as 'lead pipe' rigidity; it is present to the same extent throughout the range of movement and occurs when flexing or extending the limb. It is not affected by how fast the limb is moved. It tends to become more prominent when the patient voluntarily moves the other limb. This effect ('Froment's manoeuvre') is also called 'synkinesis'
- **Tremor**: the typical parkinsonian tremor is a rest tremor. The tremor often involves the thumb, and it is the rhythmic flexion movement of the thumb against the index finger that gives rise to the phrase 'pill-rolling'. When tremor is combined with rigidity, e.g. at the wrist, movement of the limb when the patient is relaxed will produce a feeling that the limb is stiff and moves in little jumps, like a cogwheel. This is the meaning of the phrase 'cogwheel rigidity'
- **Postural and gait disturbance**: the typical parkinsonian gait is described as 'festinant', which literally means hurrying. Patients usually walk with small shuffling steps, and they have reduced arm swing. Turning round is often difficult and is achieved with multiple small steps. Postural instability may occur and can result in falls. Posture is usually flexed forward, sometimes markedly so ('camptocormia'). During walking, some patients find that their feet suddenly seem stuck to the floor, and they cannot move. This is called 'freezing'.

## Causes of parkinsonism

Table 3.1 gives a list of the causes of parkinsonism, also called 'akinetic–rigid syndromes'. This may appear to be a rather daunting list at first sight, but many of these conditions are rare and can be excluded from the differential diagnosis just by taking a history and examining the patient. This chapter deals with PD, with other causes of parkinsonism covered in Chapter 4.

**Table 3.1** Causes of parkinsonism

| | |
|---|---|
| Primary degenerative causes of parkinsonism | Parkinson's disease (sporadic and genetic forms) |
| | Dementia with Lewy bodies (DLB) |
| | Progressive supranuclear palsy (PSP) |
| | Multiple system atrophy (MSA) |
| | Corticobasal degeneration (CBD) |
| | Alzheimer's disease (AD) |
| | Huntington's disease (HD) |
| | Parkinsonism–amyotrophic lateral sclerosis–dementia complex of Guam |
| | Fronto-temporal dementia with parkinsonism linked to chromosome 17 (FTDP-17) |
| | Lubag (X-linked dystonia parkinsonism) |
| | Basal ganglia calcification (Fahr's syndrome) |
| | Fragile X tremor ataxia syndrome (FXTAS) |
| | Dopa-responsive dystonia (DRD) |
| | Neuroacanthocytosis (NA) |
| | Dentatorubropallidoluysian atrophy (DRPLA) |
| | Neuronal brain iron accumulation (NBIA) syndromes |
| | Spinocerebellar ataxias (esp. SCA3) |
| | Pallidal degeneration syndromes (e.g. Kufor–Rakeb disease) |
| | Neuronal intranuclear inclusion disease |
| | Neurofilament inclusion body disease |
| | Rapid-onset dystonia parkinsonism (RODP) |
| Secondary causes of parkinsonism | Drugs (esp. dopamine receptor-blocking drugs) |
| | Toxins (e.g. manganese, MPTP) |
| | Cerebrovascular disease |
| | Post-encephalitic (e.g. encephalitis lethargica, Japanese B encephalitis) |
| | Neurosyphilis |
| | Anoxic brain injury |
| | Traumatic brain injury (dementia pugilistica) |
| | Basal ganglia lesions (esp. involving the substantia nigra) |
| | Metabolic disorders (e.g. Wilson's disease, GM1 gangliosidosis) |
| | Causes of basal ganglia calcification (e.g. hypoparathyroidism) |
| | Hydrocephalus |

# Approach to the patient with parkinsonism

## History

- **Age at onset**: mean age of onset of PD is about 60. Less than 5% of those with PD have onset under 40.
- **Occupation**: any exposure risk to toxins, e.g. manganese in miners, pesticides in farmers.
- **Ethnic background**: esp. Filipino (Lubag) or Ashkenazi Jewish or North African Berber origin (*LRRK2* gene mutation commoner).
- **Character of onset**: acute or gradual.
- Any precipitant at (or close to) onset, e.g. stroke, infection, hypoxia, toxin exposure.
- **Progression**: static course, rapid progression, gradual progression.
- **Family history**: if positive, what is the mode of inheritance?
- **Drug history**: esp. exposure to dopamine receptor-blocking drugs (DRBs).
- **Pattern of parkinsonian motor symptoms**.
  - Asymmetric?
  - Is tremor present? If so, is it a typical rest tremor? Is tremor the dominant clinical feature?
  - Are the legs the main part of the body affected—'lower body parkinsonism'?
  - Is there postural instability and gait disturbance (PIGD)? If so, how soon did this develop after the onset of other symptoms?
  - Is there diurnal fluctuation of symptoms—'sleep benefit'?
- **Higher mental functions**: evidence of dementia, personality change, hallucinations, paranoid ideation, depression.
- **Sleep disturbance**: rapid eye movement (REM)-sleep behaviour disorder (RBD; ➔ p. 298), periodic limb movements of sleep (PLMS; ➔ p. 295), daytime somnolence.
- **Autonomic failure**: symptoms of orthostatic hypotension (postural dizziness, 'coat-hanger' pain), urinary urgency, frequency, incontinence, or incomplete bladder emptying, impotence.
- **Other movement disorders**: does the patient have a history consistent with additional movement disorders, e.g. dystonia, myoclonus, chorea?
- **Other neurological symptoms**, e.g. difficulty with tool use (apraxia), 'alien limb' phenomena, sensory disturbance, epilepsy, neuropathy, dysphagia, stridor.

## Examination

A 'head-to-toe' examination scheme for patients with parkinsonism is provided in Box 3.1. It is not designed to replace a full neurological and systemic examination but is instead a reminder of the important clinical signs to look for in parkinsonian patients (📽 see Video 3.1: PD writing).

### Box 3.1 Neurological examinations for patients with parkinsonism

#### Head
- Observe for reduced facial expression (facial hypomimia or 'mask-like' face), reduced blink rate, frontalis overactivity (common in progressive supranuclear palsy; ⊃ p. 96).
- Check eye movements and saccades. Look in particular for square-wave jerks, limitation of vertical movement (esp. downgaze), and slowing of vertical saccades or difficulty and delay launching saccades (oculomotor apraxia). If limitation of vertical movement, perform 'doll's eye' manoeuvre (⊃ p. 96).
- Listen to speech and breathing (hypophonic (quiet) speech, stridor, inspiratory sighing).
- Assess the neck for rigidity.

#### Limbs
- Assess for rigidity—is it asymmetric?
- Assess for resting and postural tremor (for method, see ⊃ p. 126).
- Look for bradykinesia, and note any asymmetry. There are a number of methods.
  - For the arms, look for asymmetrically reduced shoulder shrug; tap thumb and forefinger together, open and close fist, or pronate and supinate the arms, performing the movement *as fast and with as large an amplitude as possible*.
  - For the legs, ask the patient while sitting to tap the feet or lift the leg up and down and stamp the foot on the ground *as fast and with as large an amplitude as possible*.
- Look for cerebellar signs: dysmetria, dysdiadochokinesia, rebound, ataxia.

#### Gait
- Watch the patient stand—are they able to do this unassisted?
- Note the posture: flexed, anterocollis, leaning to the side?
- Assess gait initiation, step size, arm swing, presence of freezing.
- Assess ability to turn round—do they need multiple steps to do this?
- Assess heel–toe walking for ten steps.
- Assess postural stability. With the patient standing facing you, with their feet slightly apart, explain that you will give them a pull towards you and that they should try to keep their balance. After a count of three, pull the patient firmly towards you by the shoulders. Then perform the same manoeuvre from behind the patient.

#### Other
- Check blood pressure with the patient lying, and after standing for 3 minutes.
- Observe temperature and skin colour of extremities.
- Perform a cognitive assessment; check handwriting.

# Parkinson's disease

## Historical aspects
James Parkinson (1755–1824) seems an unlikely person to have described the disease that now bears his name. He was a surgeon, working most of his life in a surgery and apothecary practice in Hoxton Square London, which was established by his father. He was a political radical, supporting the French Revolution and universal suffrage, and was even examined before the royal court on suspicion of involvement in a plot to murder King George III. Apart from politics, he was a keen geologist and fossil collector. He wrote one of the first popular books on fossils and was a founding member of the Geological Society of London.

His scientific work included one of the first recognized descriptions of appendicitis and a treatise on gout. The now famous *Essay on the Shaking Palsy* was published in 1817 and contained the details of six patients whom Parkinson appears to have, in general, simply come across in the street. One of these he 'only observed at a distance', and clinical details are scanty in most of the cases. However, he uses these cases to bring together existing knowledge on tremors occurring in older people, differentiates the shaking palsy from other causes of tremor, and gives a description of the shaking palsy as a mixture of tremor, slowness, and gait disturbance, as well as non-motor features.

Parkinson's publication of the essay was not of any significant immediate impact. It was Charcot in the mid-nineteenth century who added rigidity to the signs identified by Parkinson and who first used the term 'Parkinson's disease'.

## Epidemiology
- Prevalence in the whole population is about 150 per 100 000 in the United Kingdom (UK).
- Prevalence rises steeply with age, so that it affects 300–500 per 100 000 over the age of 80.
- Lifetime risk of developing PD is about 1 in 40.
- PD occurs worldwide, but, as it is mainly a disease of older people, its prevalence is higher in countries with higher life expectancy.
- Mean age at onset is 60. Young-onset PD (onset <40 years) accounts for less than 5% of cases.
- Prevalence is slightly higher in men than women.
- Epidemiological studies have found weak associations between PD and well-water drinking, pesticide exposure, farming, and rural dwelling.
- There is a negative association between PD and smoking that is not accounted for by smokers dying younger, and therefore being less likely to develop a condition that is commoner in old age.
- There are genetic risk factors for developing PD. Overall, there is a 2.5–3 times risk of developing PD if one has a first-degree relative with PD. However, this risk changes significantly, depending on the age at onset of PD in the relative.
- In monozygotic twins, PD with onset below age 40 is associated with a high risk of PD in the other twin, but with only a 10% risk if PD occurred after age 50, similar to the rate in dizygotic twins.

# Pathophysiology of Parkinson's disease

## Pathology of Parkinson's disease
- The pathological hallmarks of PD are the presence of Lewy bodies and loss of pigmented (dopaminergic) neurons in pigmented brainstem nuclei.
- Lewy bodies are inclusions within the cytoplasm of neurons that are composed of alpha-synuclein, as well as other proteins, including ubiquitin and neurofilament protein.
- In PD, Lewy bodies are found in the basal ganglia, brainstem, and cortex, and their number correlates with disease progression.
- It is hypothesized that PD may arise through a change in the alpha-synuclein protein (caused by genetic and/or environmental factors) which makes the protein toxic and form aggregates within the cell. The response of the cell is to attempt to reduce the toxicity of the alpha-synuclein aggregates by confining them within Lewy bodies. This process is clearly not foolproof, and, when it fails, neuronal death occurs. An excess of normal wild-type alpha-synuclein can also cause PD with Lewy bodies when its gene is duplicated or triplicated.
- Damage to the substantia nigra is recognized as a hallmark of PD and is probably the major cause of motor symptoms.
- Neurodegeneration happens elsewhere in the brain in PD and may precede damage to the substantia nigra. The neuropathologist Braak has suggested that pathological changes which occur in PD can be divided into six stages—the 'Braak hypothesis'.
  - Stages 1 and 2: pathology is confined to certain structures in the brainstem, but not yet the substantia nigra
  - Stages 3 and 4: pathology spreads to the midbrain and basal ganglia
  - Stages 5 and 6: changes spread to the cortex.
- This may explain the onset of sleep disturbance and loss of sense of smell prior to the onset of motor symptoms, as well as other 'non-motor' symptoms of PD (➔ p. 36).

## Basal ganglia circuits and Parkinson's disease
- With the basal ganglia circuits outlined in Chapter 2 in mind (➔ p. 18), it is possible to see how the damage that occurs to the substantia nigra in PD could cause a decrease in movement.
- The SNc sends out dopaminergic neurons which have a positive effect via D1 receptors on the direct 'go' pathway, and a negative effect via D2 receptors on the indirect 'stop' pathway.
- Therefore, if activity from the SNc is reduced due to degeneration of dopaminergic neurons, the activity of the direct pathway will tend to decrease, and the activity of the indirect pathway will tend to increase. This combination will increase the amount of inhibition from the basal ganglia on the motor cortex.

- As discussed in Chapter 2, there are problems with these simple models of basal ganglia circuits. However, they provide a rationale for the effectiveness of dopamine in the treatment of PD, which is hypothesized to reset the balance between direct and indirect pathway activity.
- Emphasis has now shifted to the importance of excessively synchronized neuronal firing within the motor circuit at the beta frequency (12–20 Hz). Suppression of this activity is associated with initiation of movement or change in movement pattern in healthy people. It is suggested that, in PD, excessive synchrony at this frequency causes difficulty in initiating and maintaining movement. It is of note that levodopa and DBS reduce beta synchrony.

## Parkinson's disease: history

Most of the important aspects of history taking in PD are covered in the section on the approach to parkinsonism (→ p. 4). Some further specific points regarding PD are:
- Patients with PD have two common presentations: (1) presentation with asymmetric tremor as the main symptom/sign, or (2) presentation with asymmetric bradykinesia and rigidity as the main symptoms/signs.
- The history of those with tremor is usually that of an insidious onset of tremor in one hand, often first noticed by a family member, rather than the patient, and gradually worsening, eventually prompting the patient to seek advice.
- In those with prominent bradykinesia and rigidity, the presentation can be more varied. Patients often complain of aching in one limb, stiffness, weakness, or even loss of coordination. The appropriate referral of these patients is often delayed, or mis-referral occurs.
- On direct questioning, patients with PD often report other symptoms, some of which may have begun some time before the motor symptoms that have prompted the referral. It is essential to ask about these symptoms, as they often cause more disability than the major motor symptoms:
  - sleep disturbance, e.g. PLMS (→ p. 295), RBD (→ p. 298), daytime somnolence
  - inability or difficulty in turning over in bed
  - depression
  - fatigue, apathy, loss of motivation
  - loss of sense of smell
  - excessive sweating
  - pain in a limb
  - abnormal postures (sometimes painful) in a limb.
- It is essential to understand the functional impact of all symptoms, and which symptoms are having the most important effect on the quality of life.

There are a number of 'red flags' that may suggest atypical parkinsonism, rather than PD, and these should be specifically addressed during history taking:

- **cognitive decline and behavioural change**: in particular, visual hallucinations, fluctuation in mental performance throughout the day
- **autonomic disturbance**: postural hypotension, urinary symptoms, impotence
- falls
- sudden onset and/or stepwise deterioration
- history of dopamine receptor-blocking drug use.

# Parkinson's disease: examination

Most of the important aspects of examination in PD are covered in the section on the approach to parkinsonism (→ p. 24). However, some further specific points regarding PD are given.

- Bedside testing of eye movements and saccades in PD is normal. Many normal older people have a limitation of upgaze, which does not improve with a doll's eye manoeuvre (→ p. 24).
- This should not be misinterpreted as pathological supranuclear gaze palsy.
- A number of different tremors can occur in PD (for a full description, see → p. 128), including:
  - asymmetric 3–4 Hz rest tremor of the arms or legs. If affecting the arms, it often involves the thumb and forefinger (pill-rolling)
  - asymmetric 6 Hz postural tremor which occurs immediately on stretching out the arms
  - asymmetric 3–4 Hz tremor which occurs a few seconds after the arms are outstretched (re-emergent tremor)
  - jaw tremor
  - tongue tremor
- Head tremor is very unusual in PD and should lead to careful reconsideration of the diagnosis.

There are a number of 'red flags' on examination which suggest atypical parkinsonism, rather than PD, and should form part of the examination of all patients with suspected PD (📹 see Video 3.2: PD gait):

- eye movement disorder
- early marked postural instability, falls, dysphagia, dysarthria
- cerebellar signs
- prominent severe gait disturbance, without significant parkinsonian signs in the arms
- significant postural drop in blood pressure (>30 mmHg) not due to drugs
- presence of other movement disorders (although dystonia may occur in genetic or sporadic PD, particularly if young onset).

## Parkinson's disease: clinical diagnosis

There is no diagnostic test for PD, and it remains a clinical diagnosis. There are some tests that can assist in the differential diagnosis of PD (➔ p. 40), but, even in specialist movement disorder clinics with access to such investigations, the error rate in diagnosis ranges from 10% to 20%. The commonest alternative diagnoses are ET, drug-induced parkinsonism, dystonic tremor, vascular parkinsonism, progressive supranuclear palsy (PSP), multiple system atrophy (MSA), and corticobasal degeneration (CBD).

A set of well-validated criteria (the UK Parkinson's Disease Society Brain Bank Clinical Criteria) exist to assist in the clinical diagnosis of PD and have a specificity and sensitivity of 98.1% and 90.4%, respectively (Box 3.2). They bring together many of the aspects of history taking and examination.

## Box 3.2 UK Parkinson's Disease Society Brain Bank Clinical Criteria for the diagnosis of Parkinson's disease

*Step 1. Diagnosis of parkinsonian syndrome*

Patients must have bradykinesia (as defined on ➲ p. 22) plus at least one of the following:
- muscular rigidity
- 4–6 Hz rest tremor
- postural instability not caused by primary visual, vestibular, cerebellar, or proprioceptive dysfunction.

*Step 2. Exclusion criteria for Parkinson's disease*

Patients must not have any of the following:
- history of repeated strokes with stepwise progression of parkinsonian features
- history of repeated head injury
- history of definite encephalitis
- oculogyric crises
- neuroleptic treatment at onset of symptoms
- more than one affected relative
- sustained remission
- strictly unilateral features after 3 years
- supranuclear gaze palsy
- cerebellar signs
- early severe autonomic involvement
- early severe dementia with disturbances of memory, language, and praxis
- Babinski sign
- presence of a cerebral tumour or communicating hydrocephalus
- negative response to large doses of levodopa in the absence of malabsorption
- MPTP exposure.

*Step 3. Supportive prospective positive criteria for Parkinson's disease*

Three or more required for diagnosis of definite Parkinson's disease, in combination with step 1:
- unilateral onset
- rest tremor present
- progressive disorder
- persistent asymmetry affecting side of onset most
- excellent response (70–100%) to levodopa
- severe levodopa-induced chorea
- levodopa response for 5 years or more
- clinical course of 10 years or more.

Reproduced from *J Neurol Neurosurg Psychiatry*, **55**, Hughes AJ et al., Accuracy of clinical diagnosis of idiopathic Parkinson's disease: a clinico-pathological study of 100 cases. pp. 181–4, Copyright (1992), with permission from BMJ Publishing Group Ltd.

# Non-motor symptoms in Parkinson's disease: dementia

## Introduction
Dementia is a common occurrence in PD. After 10 years of symptoms, nearly 80% of patients will have dementia. In many, this is mild and not severely disabling. However, in others, dementia can be severe. Severe dementia predicts entry into residential care and increases mortality.

## Mild cognitive impairment in non-demented Parkinson's disease patients
Around 25% of non-demented PD patients have mild cognitive impairment (PD-MCI). The frequency of PD-MCI increases with age, disease duration, and disease severity. Impairments may be identified on neuropsychological testing and can have an impact on performance in daily life. The common deficits that are found include slowness of thought and reasoning, poor recall, and difficulty in changing cognitive strategies when faced with new tasks (cognitive inflexibility). PD-MCI is a risk factor to develop PD dementia, and formal clinical criteria for PD-MCI have been developed.

## Dementia and Parkinson's disease
Dementia occurs in PD, either as a consequence of the pathological process underlying PD itself (dementia with Lewy bodies (DLB), Parkinson's disease-associated dementia (PDD)) or as an additional pathological process causing dementia (e.g. PD with Alzheimer's disease, PD with vascular dementia). Age is the most prominent risk factor to develop PDD, independently of the age of PD onset. The risk to develop PDD correlates with the severity of motor signs, the presence of visual hallucinations, the PD phenotype (e.g. prominent axial rigidity and bradykinesia, as opposed to tremor), and the presence of mild cognitive impairment.

### Dementia with Lewy bodies and Parkinson's disease-associated dementia
- Although there is still debate, DLB and PDD are probably two ends of the same spectrum of disorder and are both characterized by Lewy body deposition in the cerebral cortex.
- DLB is a very common form of dementia.
- Both DLB and PDD cause a similar pattern of impairment:

- fluctuating level of alertness, attention, and cognition
- visual hallucinations: these are often of people or animals, and are usually worse in the evening
- parkinsonism (often without prominent tremor)
- REM-sleep behaviour disorder (RBD; ➔ p. 298)
- falls
- sensitivity to dopamine receptor-blocking drugs (DRBs): even atypical DRBs cause severe parkinsonism in patients with DLB, in contrast to patients with Alzheimer's disease.

In order to diagnose DLB, cognitive impairment must occur prior to, or within the first year of, parkinsonian symptoms. PDD has similar symptoms but simply occurs later in the course of PD. Short-term memory is less affected by DLB and PDD than it is in Alzheimer's disease. Both DLB and PDD are treated in the same manner, as discussed on ➔ p. 68.

# Other non-motor symptoms in Parkinson's disease

Apart from dementia, a number of further non-motor symptoms can occur (Table 3.2) and are a common source of disability in PD. Many patients do not spontaneously volunteer information about these symptoms, and specific questions regarding them should form part of the routine assessment of patients with PD. Treatment of these symptoms can be difficult but is as important as treatment of motor symptoms, and is discussed on ➔ p. 68. Even if treatment is not possible, many patients gain benefit from acknowledgement of these symptoms and an explanation that they are due to PD.

Table 3.2 Non-motor symptoms in Parkinson's disease

| | |
|---|---|
| Neuropsychiatric | Dementia |
| | Depression |
| | Apathy |
| | Abulia |
| | Anxiety |
| | Loss of libido |
| Autonomic | Constipation |
| | Urinary incontinence |
| | Erectile dysfunction |
| | Excessive sweating |
| | Postural hypotension |
| | Excessive salivation |
| Sleep disturbance | REM sleep behaviour disorder |
| | Periodic limb movements of sleep |
| | Vivid dreams |
| | Daytime somnolence |
| Sensory symptoms | Pain |
| | Paraesthesiae |
| Other | Fatigue |
| | Loss of sense of smell |

Other non-motor symptoms can occur as a complication of therapy and are discussed on ➔ p. 74.

# Parkinson's disease: investigations

PD is a clinical diagnosis, and investigations are not necessary for the majority of patients. However, where there is doubt regarding the diagnosis, certain investigations may be helpful.

## Levodopa challenge

A hallmark of PD is the response of motor symptoms to dopaminergic drugs such as levodopa. Therefore, a beneficial response to a single dose of levodopa has been viewed, *incorrectly*, as a diagnostic test for PD. This test has the advantage of being quick, cheap, and widely available, but has a number of problems.

- Some patients with PD do not respond to single doses of levodopa and require sustained high-dose treatment to obtain benefit.
- Some atypical parkinsonian conditions, including MSA, PSP, and vascular parkinsonism, may initially respond to levodopa.
- Other factors, such as poor absorption of levodopa, inadequate clinical skills/inappropriate protocol to assess benefit, and placebo effect, may affect the result of a levodopa challenge.

Lack of effect from a levodopa challenge does not automatically mean that the patient is levodopa-unresponsive. Lack of response to a dose of approximately 1000 mg/day of levodopa given for at least 2 months is much more meaningful. A protocol for performing a levodopa challenge is given in Box 3.3.

Note that recent National Institute for Health and Care Excellence (NICE) guidelines (http://www.nice.org.uk) specifically state that a levodopa challenge should *not* be used in the differential diagnosis of a parkinsonian condition.

## Imaging

- **Structural (magnetic resonance imaging (MRI)/computerized tomography (CT))**: normal in PD. Definitely abnormal in some conditions causing atypical parkinsonism (e.g. tumour, hydrocephalus). Abnormalities on MRI can occur in conditions commonly confused with PD (e.g. PSP, MSA) but are not always present.
- **Diffusion-weighted imaging (DWI)**: DWI is an MRI technique which can identify differences in the diffusivity of water molecules in different parts of the brain. Striatal increase in the DWI signal is seen in PSP and MSA, but not in PD. Although still a research tool, DWI is a widely available MRI technique which may in the future help differentiate PD from some atypical parkinsonian conditions.
- **Single-photon emission computerized tomography (SPECT)**: tracers (e.g. beta-CIT, FP-CIT), which bind to the dopamine transporter protein (DAT) in the nigrostriatal nerve endings, show a reduction in binding in PD which has some correlation with disease progression. However, these 'DAT scans' are also abnormal in PSP, MSA, and CBD. They are typically normal in drug-induced parkinsonism and ET.

- **Positron emission tomography (PET)**: less widely available than SPECT scans. The binding of fluorine-18-labelled dopa is reduced in PD and parallels disease progression to some extent. Like SPECT scans, PET scans are also abnormal in PSP, MSA, and CBD.
- **Transcranial sonography**: transcranial B-mode ultrasonography can reveal reduced echogenicity of the substantia nigra in patients with PD. It is still a research tool, but it may be a simple and cheap method to support the diagnosis of PD and differentiate it from causes of atypical parkinsonism.

### Other investigations

- **Olfactory testing**: over 90% of patients with PD develop impairment of the sense of smell, and this is usually an early feature of the disease. It is much less common in MSA and PSP. Olfactory dysfunction is also very uncommon in young-onset parkinsonism due to parkin gene mutations.
- **Genetic testing**: although a number of genes for PD have been described (→ p. 38), they are not relevant in the investigation of most patients with suspected PD. In patients with young-onset disease or with a strong family history, particularly in Ashkenazi Jews or patients from North Africa, genetic testing for parkin or LRRK2 may be appropriate (→ p. 44).

---

**Box 3.3 How to perform a levodopa challenge**

- If the patient is not already treated with dopaminergic drugs, pretreat for at least 24 hours with 20 mg of domperidone three times daily (tds).
- Avoid high-protein meals immediately prior to the challenge.
- Assess the patient immediately prior to the challenge:
  - Administer the motor section of the MDS Unified Parkinson's Disease Rating Scale (MDS-UPDRS)
  - Place two markers, 30 cm apart, on a table in front of the patient, and ask them to place their index finger on one of the markers. Ask the patient to move their finger between the markers ten times as quickly as possible, and use a stopwatch to time how long they take. Repeat with the other hand
  - Time how long it takes the patient to walk 10 m.
- Give two tablets of co-beneldopa 25/100 dispersible in water.
- Repeat the same assessments after 0.5 hour and 1 hour, and calculate the percentage improvement. ~25% improvement is considered a positive challenge.

# Genetics of Parkinson's disease

Most patients with PD have apparently sporadic disease, without a clear family history. Although the overall risk of developing PD if one has a first-degree relative with PD is 2.5–3 times the normal risk, this is very dependent on age at onset. In people with a first-degree relative with onset over 65, the risk of PD is broadly similar to that in the general population. In those with a first-degree relative with onset under 40, the chance of developing PD is significantly higher.

## Genes in Parkinson's disease

To date, 20 loci have been identified in familial PD (*PARK1–20*), and 13 genes have been identified. The PARK designations refer to monogenic forms of autosomal dominant typical PD (*PARK1/4, PARK5, PARK8, PARK17, PARK18*), autosomal recessive PD (*PARK2, PARK6, PARK7*), autosomal recessive atypical parkinsonism (*PARK9, PARK14–15, PARK19–20*), and susceptibility loci (*PARK3, PARK10–13, PARK16*) (Box 3.4).

### Box 3.4 Autosomal dominant Parkinson's disease

#### PARK1/PARK4: alpha-synuclein

- Historically important genetic cause of PD, as it turned the spotlight on alpha-synuclein as a potentially important protein in the pathogenesis of PD.
- Numerically unimportant as a cause of dominant PD, estimated higher prevalence in Greece.
- Duplications of the gene tend to cause disease similar to sporadic PD with onset in the 40s to 60s, whereas triplications (*PARK4*) cause younger-onset disease, often with dementia.

#### PARK5: ubiquitin C-terminal ligase 1 (UCHL1)

- Mutation only reported in one family with onset of PD in the 50s.

#### PARK8: leucine-rich repeat kinase 2 (LRRK2)

- Commonest cause of dominantly inherited PD.
- LRRK2 is a protein kinase, but currently its function is unknown.
- Causes a clinical picture similar to sporadic PD, with onset in the 50s or 60s.
- Pathology is remarkably variable, with most patients reported showing Lewy bodies, but others nigral degeneration without Lewy bodies, and even tau pathology similar to PSP.
- *LRRK2* mutations may account for up to 1% of apparently sporadic PD cases.
- In the Ashkenazi Jewish and North African populations, it may account for about 13% of sporadic cases, and 30% of those with a positive family history.

### PARK3, PARK10, PARK11 (GIGYF2), PARK12, PARK13 (HTRA2), PARK16 (RAB7L1)
- Susceptibility loci and genes.

### PARK17: vacuolar protein sorting 35 (VPS35)
- A rare cause of late-onset, levodopa-responsive parkinsonism, with mean age of onset of 51 years.
- Very few kindreds described.
- There is still no pathology available.

### PARK18: eukaryotic translation initiation factor 4-gamma 1 (EIF4G1)
- A rare cause of mild, late-onset, levodopa-responsive parkinsonism, with mean age of onset of 64 years.
- Very few kindreds described.
- Pathology showed diffuse Lewy body disease.

## Autosomal recessive Parkinson's disease
### PARK2: parkin
- A common cause of autosomal recessive PD. Mutations present in up to 65% of those with juvenile-onset PD (<20 years) and about 20% of those with young-onset PD (<40 years), rising to 50% if a positive family history is present.
- Parkin is a ubiquitin ligase, and dysfunction is predicted to interfere with ubiquitination, and therefore clearance of toxic proteins.
- Typical age at onset is in the 30s.
- Limb dystonia is often prominent, together with subtle upper motor neuron-like signs. Psychiatric disturbance may occur. This phenotype is similar to some patients with dopa-responsive dystonia (DRD) (➔ p. 210).
- Parkin-associated PD is levodopa-responsive. Generally, disease progression is very slow.
- Pathology shows nigral degeneration, but typically no Lewy bodies.
- Most patients are compound heterozygotes (two different mutations, one on each gene). Heterozygotes can develop PD, usually with onset in the 60s or 70s.

### PARK6: PTEN-induced kinase 1 (PINK1)
- A rare cause of recessive PD.
- Onset typically in the 30s or 40s.
- *PINK1* encodes a mitochondrial protein of unknown function.

### PARK7: oncogene DJ-1 (DJ-1)
- A rare cause of recessive PD.
- Onset typically in the 30s or 40s.
- The protein encoded by *DJ-1* appears to play a role in response to oxidative stress. Autosomal recessive atypical parkinsonism.

*(Continued)*

### PARK 9: ATPase type 132 (ATP13A2, Kufor–Rakeb)
- A very rare cause of recessive levodopa-responsive parkinsonism.
- Rapidly progressive juvenile-onset parkinsonism described with supranuclear gaze palsy, spasticity, dystonia, dementia, myoclonus. Loss-of-function mutations have been described in the *ATP13A2* gene, which encodes a mainly neuronal P-type ATPase.
- Pathology of ceroid lipofuscinosis.

### PARK 14: phospholipase A2, group 6 (PLA2G6)
- Rare cause of complicated, variable response to levodopa, juvenile dystonia–parkinsonism–spasticity syndrome.
- Lewy body pathology.

### PARK 15: F-box only protein 7 (FBXO7)
- Rare cause of complicated, variable response to levodopa, juvenile dystonia–parkinsonism–spasticity syndrome.

### PARK 19: DnaJ homolog, subfamily C, member 6 (DNAJC6) and PARK 20: synaptojanin 1 (SYNJ1)
- Rare causes of complicated, juvenile, poorly levodopa-responsive parkinsonism with dystonia and cognitive dysfunction.

## Risk genes in Parkinson's disease
A number of genes and loci are associated with risk for PD (Box 3.4). Disease risk may be associated with allelic variants of known genes such as *SNCA* and *LRRK2*. The *LRRK2* p.G2385R variant is common in Asian populations and approximately doubles the risk for PD, while the *SNCA* promoter region REP-1 polymorphism is associated with a 1.4-fold increased risk. Heterozygous mutations in the glucocerebrosidase (*GBA*) gene convey a 5-fold increased risk to develop PD, arguing that this may be a dominant form with reduced penetrance and suggesting that PD and Gaucher's disease (caused by *GBA* homozygous mutations) might share common underlying molecular mechanisms. The number of genetic risk factors identified is continuously expanding and now includes over 20 independent loci.

## Genetic testing in Parkinson's disease
Genetic testing is not indicated in patients with typical sporadic PD. In those with a dominant family history and Ashkenazi Jewish or North African origin, testing for *LRRK2* mutations can be considered, while, in those with a dominant family history and Greek origin, testing for *SCNA* mutations can be considered. In those with young-onset PD, with or without a family history, testing for parkin mutations can be considered. No specific treatments exist for those with identified mutations causing PD, other than those available for all patients with PD. However, identification of gene mutations can be helpful in genetic counselling of patients, which is much more important for dominant than recessive genes.

# Breaking the news

In stark contrast to many degenerative diseases of the nervous system, PD is a treatable condition which often has a fairly benign course for a number of years. However, the public perception of PD is usually very different, and the diagnosis of PD can have a devastating psychological impact on the patient.

## Diagnosis
- If possible, it is preferable to have a family member/close friend present if the patient agrees.
- Ask the patient if they have had any thoughts on the possible diagnosis. They will have often considered PD, and this provides a good place from which to start the discussion.
- Explain that you think that the most likely diagnosis is PD and that this diagnosis is based on the clinical features because there are no diagnostic tests for PD.
- Explain that PD is a very common condition and that it is not curable but is treatable.
- Explain that symptoms may slowly become worse over time but that, with treatment, many patients remain mildly affected and can carry on entirely normal lives.

## Treatment
- Explain that treatment is symptomatic, and therefore the choice of when to start treatment depends on the patient's assessment of their degree of disability.
- Explain that there is a range of treatment options and that, over time, more treatment is needed to control symptoms adequately.
- Often discussion of treatment is best left to a follow-up visit, by which time the patient may have had an opportunity to read up a little about the condition.

## Other issues
- Explain the plan for follow-up of the patient, and explain the role and method of contact of the PD nurse specialist (PDNS) (if one is available).
- Explain that a diagnosis of PD does not prohibit driving (unless there are other factors such as dementia), but patients should inform the driving licence authority and, as a precautionary measure, their driving insurance company of the diagnosis.
- Give literature and/or contact details of PD patient support organizations, if wanted. Caution against the large amount of dubious information on PD available from the Internet and other sources.

## Management of Parkinson's disease

The main thrust of the following sections on management of PD is on medications, but this does not mean that successful management of PD is solely a case of dispensing the right drug at the right time. Management of PD is based on a long-term relationship with the patient, and it is the quality of this relationship that is of the greatest importance in the successful management of patients with PD.

### Multidisciplinary management of Parkinson's disease

Management of PD within a multidisciplinary team is particularly important. This does not mean that every patient needs to be seen by each member of the team in a kind of 'one size fits all' merry-go-round of appointments with different doctors and therapists. This is not only a waste of time for the patient, but also leads to the patient feeling that no one is actually in control of their treatment. The best sort of multi-disciplinary arrangement is a team that can respond quickly to the needs of a particular patient at a particular time. At one stage, the neurologist may be leading the consultations and follow-up; at another stage, the PD specialist nurse may be primarily involved, and, at yet another stage, psychiatric input may be the most important intervention. The key aspect of this sort of team is a coordinated approach which allows the appropriate therapist to be accessed by the patient in a timely and well-organized fashion. Members of such a multidisciplinary team could include:

- PDNS
- neurologist/geriatrician
- psychiatrist
- physiotherapist
- occupational therapist
- speech and language therapist
- clinic organizer/personal assistant
- neurosurgeon
- disability benefits/social services adviser
- neuropsychologist
- counsellor.

### Medical treatment of Parkinson's disease

The following pages deal with the different medical treatments available for PD and discuss at some length the currently unresolved controversies regarding when to initiate treatment for motor symptoms and which drugs to use.

Within this complex debate, it is easy to lose sight of the fact that non-motor symptoms, such as depression, urinary disturbance, fatigue, and apathy, are a major contribution to the overall burden of disability in PD. In contrast to motor symptoms, there is much less evidence regarding how non-motor symptoms should be treated. However, successful treatment is possible for some symptoms and can have a major impact on quality of life. Even if treatment is not possible, a simple explanation that these symptoms are part of PD can be very helpful for patients and their families.

## National Institute for Health and Care Excellence guidelines for Parkinson's disease

NICE is a government-funded body within the UK which assesses and publishes guidelines on the management of medical conditions within the National Health Service (NHS). PD was the subject of a NICE review in 2006, and the comprehensive report, together with supporting literature, is available online at http://www.nice.org.uk.

The major recommendations of this review are as follows.

- People with suspected PD should be referred quickly and untreated to a specialist with expertise in the differential diagnosis of the condition. Patients should be seen within 6 weeks, or within 2 weeks for later-stage/complex problems.
- The diagnosis of PD should be reviewed regularly and reconsidered if atypical clinical features develop. Patients with PD should be seen every 6–12 months.
- Acute levodopa/apomorphine challenges should not be used in the differential diagnosis of parkinsonian syndromes.
- People with PD should have regular access to the following, which may be provided by a PDNS:
  - clinical monitoring and medication adjustment
  - a continuing point of contact for support, including home visits when appropriate
  - a reliable source of information about clinical and social matters of concern to people with PD and their carers
- Physiotherapy should be available for people with PD. Particular consideration should be given to gait re-education, improvement of balance and flexibility, enhancement of aerobic capacity, improvement of movement initiation, improvement of functional independence, including mobility and activities of daily living, and provision of advice regarding safety in the home environment.
- Occupational therapy should be available for people with PD. Particular consideration should be given to: maintenance of work and family roles, home care and leisure activities, improvement and maintenance of transfers and mobility, improvement of personal self-care such as eating, drinking, washing, and dressing, environmental issues to improve safety and motor function, and cognitive assessment and appropriate intervention.
- Speech and language therapy (SLT) should be available to people with PD. Particular consideration should be given to: improvement of vocal loudness and pitch range, including speech therapy programmes such as Lee Silverman Voice Treatment, teaching strategies to optimize speech intelligibility, ensuring that an effective means of communication is maintained throughout the course of the disease, including the use of assistive technologies, and review and management to support the safety and efficiency of swallowing and to minimize the risk of aspiration.
- Palliative care requirements of people with PD should be considered throughout all phases of the disease. People with PD and their carers should be given the opportunity to discuss end-of-life issues with appropriate health-care professionals.

## Treatment of motor symptoms

### Drugs available to treat motor symptoms of Parkinson's disease

Fig. 3.1 is a schematic drawing of a dopaminergic synapse, indicating the natural mechanism of dopaminergic transmission and the site of action of each of the drugs mentioned in Box 3.5. Each of these medications is discussed in detail on subsequent pages. This is followed by a discussion of the controversial area of when treatment should be initiated and with which drug.

> **Box 3.5 Drugs available to treat motor symptoms of Parkinson's disease**
> - Levodopa:
>   - co-careldopa
>   - co-beneldopa
> - Dopamine agonists:
>   - pramipexole
>   - ropinirole
>   - rotigotine
>   - cabergoline (no longer used in general clinical practice)
>   - bromocriptine (no longer used in general clinical practice)
> - Monoamine oxidase inhibitors:
>   - selegiline
>   - rasagiline
> - Catechol-*O*-methyltransferase inhibitors:
>   - entacapone
>   - tolcapone. (no longer used in general clinical practice)
> - Amantadine
> - Anticholinergics (trihexyphenidyl and others)

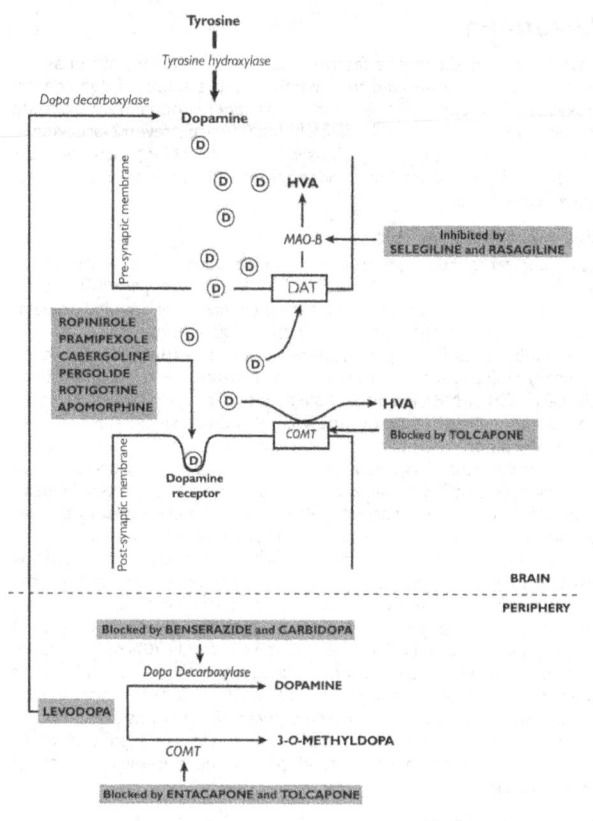

**Fig. 3.1** The dopaminergic synapse and site of action of drugs available for treatment of motor symptoms in Parkinson's disease. COMT, catechol-*O*-methyltransferase; DAT, dopamine transporter protein; HVA, homovanillic acid; MAO-B, monoamine oxidase B.

# Levodopa

Levodopa is still the most effective treatment available for motor symptoms in PD. It is converted to dopamine via the action of dopa decarboxylase. Levodopa is given with a peripheral dopa decarboxylase inhibitor (either benserazide or carbidopa) which prevents breakdown of levodopa in the periphery. Benserazide and carbidopa do not cross the blood–brain barrier, but levodopa does and is metabolized to dopamine in the brain.

## Preparations available

Levodopa prescriptions are usually written as dopa decarboxylase dose/levodopa dose, e.g. co-careldopa 25/100 = 25 mg carbidopa + 100 mg levodopa. Confusingly, doses may be combined in names of branded preparations, e.g. Sinemet® 110 = 10 mg carbidopa + 100 mg levodopa.

A number of different preparations are available (Box 3.6). As well as ordinary tablets/capsules, there are modified-release formulations (usually called CR or MR) and dispersible forms which are dissolved in water. Levodopa is absorbed across the wall of the proximal ileum and also across the blood–brain barrier by an active transport mechanism in competition with other large neutral amino acids, so some patients notice that the amino acid load derived from large amounts of protein in meals may interfere with its absorption. Standard tablets and capsules are better absorbed on an empty stomach than taken with food. However, the bottle usually says 'take with food', which is only required in those few patients in whom it causes sickness. Modified-release formulations can have a longer duration of action but may produce a rather unpredictable response, particularly in more advanced patients. The bioavailability of levodopa ingested in modified-release tablets is only 70% of the equivalent dose in ordinary tablets. Dispersible forms of levodopa have a faster onset of action than tablet forms and can be useful for situations where a rapid response is required, but tend to wear off sooner at the end of the dose. Stalevo® is a combination of entacapone and levodopa–carbidopa. Duodopa® is a formulation of levodopa–carbidopa designed for direct jejunal infusion.

## Starting levodopa*

- Start levodopa 50 mg twice daily (bd).
- Increase after 4 days to 50 mg tds.
- If required, increase the dose by 50 mg every week to reach 100 mg tds. This is a common maintenance dose with initial therapy, and patients should be reviewed on this dosage before considering further increases.
- Further increases should be performed slowly if required, usually in 50 mg increments.
- The maximum daily dose of levodopa is in the region of 1.5–2 g daily.

## Side effects

- Early in treatment, a few patients develop nausea or vomiting. These are usually well controlled by domperidone, and tolerance usually develops rapidly over a week or two.
- Less common side effects include postural hypotension, hallucinations, daytime somnolence, and sudden onset of sleep. Patients should be warned regarding sleepiness and should exercise caution with driving and operating machinery.
- Important chronic side effects include dyskinesia and on–off fluctuations, the so-called 'long-term levodopa syndrome' (➔ p. 78). These are common with chronic treatment and must be discussed with the patient before beginning levodopa treatment.
- There have been reports of reactivation of melanoma with levodopa, and therefore caution is advised, together with dermatological surveillance, in those with previous melanoma.
- Sudden withdrawal of levodopa can result in neuroleptic malignant-like syndrome (➔ p. 264).
- Peripheral neuropathy.

### Box 3.6 Available preparations of levodopa in the UK

#### Co-beneldopa (benserazide + levodopa)

*Dispersible*

- Co-beneldopa 12.5/50 (12.5 mg DDC/50 mg LD); scored
- Co-beneldopa 25/100 (25 mg DDC/100 mg LD); scored

*Capsules*

- Co-beneldopa 12.5/50 (12.5 mg DDC/50 mg LD); blue/grey capsules
- Co-beneldopa 25/100 (25 mg DDC/100 mg LD); blue/pink capsules
- Co-beneldopa 50/200 (5 0 mg DDC/200 mg LD); blue/caramel capsules
- Modified-release co-beneldopa 25/100 (25 mg DDC/100 mg LD); dark green/light blue capsules

#### Co-careldopa (carbidopa + levodopa)

*Tablets*

- Co-careldopa 12.5/50 (12.5 mg DDC/50 mg LD); yellow tablets, scored
- Co-careldopa 10/100 (10 mg DDC/100 mg LD); blue tablets, scored
- Co-careldopa 25/100 (25 mg DDC/100 mg LD); yellow tablets, scored
- Co-careldopa 25/250 (25 mg DDC/250 mg LD); blue tablets, scored

*(Continued)*

## CHAPTER 3 **Parkinson's disease**

*Modified-release*
- Co-careldopa 25/100 (25 mg DDC/100 mg LD) tablets; pink or caramel CR; orange–brown
- Co-careldopa 50/200 (50 mg DDC/200 mg LD); peach tablets, scored

### With entacapone (all preparations are brown tablets)
(➲ p. 62)
- Stalevo® 50 mg/12.5 mg/200 mg (50 mg LD/12.5 mg DDC/200 mg entacapone)
- Stalevo® 75 mg/18.75 mg/200 mg (75 mg LD/18.75 mg DDC/200 mg entacapone)
- Stalevo® 100 mg/25 mg/200 mg (100 mg LD/25 mg DDC/200 mg entacapone)
- Stalevo® 125 mg/31.25 mg/200 mg (125 mg LD/31.25 mg DDC/200 mg entacapone)
- Stalevo® 150 mg/37.5 mg/200 mg (150 mg LD/37.5 mg DDC/200 mg entacapone)
- Stalevo® 175 mg/43.75 mg/200 mg (175 mg LD/43.75 mg DDC/200 mg entacapone)
- Stalevo® 200 mg/50 mg/200 mg (200 mg LD/50 mg DDC/200 mg entacapone)

### Duodopa®
- Levodopa-carbidopa gel for direct jejunal infusion.

DDC, dopa decarboxylase inhibitor; LD, levodopa.

# Dopamine agonists: 1

Dopamine agonists directly stimulate post-synaptic dopamine receptors. A number of dopamine agonists have been developed, divided into those that have an ergoline structure (bromocriptine, lisuride, pergolide, cabergoline—the 'ergot' agonists), and those that do not (pramipexole, ropinirole, rotigotine, apomorphine—the 'non-ergots'). Dopamine agonists are effective in the treatment of motor symptoms in PD as monotherapy and are only rarely associated with the long-term side effects of dyskinesia and the on–off fluctuations seen with levodopa. However, they are less effective than levodopa and can cause catastrophic impulse control disorders (ICDs). Dopamine agonists differ in their affinity for different subtypes of dopamine receptors. The practical relevance of these differences in affinity is not certain, and there are no clear differences in efficacy between individual dopamine agonists, with the exception of apomorphine. All the dopamine agonists come in tablet form, apart from rotigotine, which is available as a skin patch, and apomorphine, which is available as a liquid for subcutaneous injection or continuous infusion through a pump (→ p. 83 and p. 84).

## Fibrosis and ergot agonists

Ergot dopamine agonists, in particular pergolide, have been associated with fibrotic reactions affecting the lung, heart, and retroperitoneal space. Although rare, these complications led to advice that, before starting ergot agonists, patients should have baseline erythrocyte sedimentation rate (ESR), creatinine, and chest X-ray, as well as clinical assessment of cardiac and respiratory function, and they should be warned of the possibility of fibrotic complications and monitored clinically during treatment for signs of dyspnoea, cough, chest pain, cardiac failure, and abdominal pain. In practice, virtually all patients on ergot agonists have been switched to non-ergot dopamine agonists.

## Side effects

- Common acute side effects are nausea, vomiting, and postural hypotension, and are usually successfully managed with domperidone, pretreatment with which can prevent or reduce initial sickness in *de novo* patients.
- Excessive sleepiness and sudden onset of sleep ('sleep attacks') can occur, and patients must be specifically warned about this and of the need to stop driving if these side effects occur.
- Hallucinations can occur with dopamine agonists, particularly in older patients.
- ICDs, including pathological gambling, compulsive shopping, hypersexuality, binge eating, and compulsive Internet use, and paranoid states, particularly in relation to suspected marital infidelity ('Othello syndrome'), between them occur in at least 13.5% of treated subjects, especially younger and male subjects with a personal or family history of addiction to smoking, alcohol, or other substances. Patients considering agonist use *must* be specifically warned of these side effects before deciding to take agonists and be interrogated about them at every visit.

- Leg swelling is a common side effect and may be severe.
- Parkinsonian symptoms often worsen in the first few weeks of therapy, as dopamine agonists stimulate D2 pre-synaptic receptors, which reduce endogenous dopamine production. This occurs before there is sufficient stimulation of post-synaptic receptors to give benefit on symptoms. Patients should be told about the possibility of this initial worsening of symptoms, and nevertheless to continue with dose escalation.

## Dopamine agonists: 2

### How to introduce different dopamine agonists

*Pramipexole*
- A non-ergot agonist with affinity for D2 and D3 receptors.
- Tablets provided: 0.125 mg salt (88 micrograms base), 0.25 mg salt (180 micrograms base), 0.5 mg salt (350 micrograms base), and 1 mg salt (700 micrograms base). Prescription was previously by amount of base in each tablet, leading to rather complex mathematics as the dose was escalated. Thankfully, prescriptions can now be written as the amount of pramipexole salt.
  - Initiated at 0.125 mg salt tds, increasing after 5–7 days to 0.25 mg salt tds, then after a further 2 weeks to 0.5 mg salt tds. Typical maintenance dose is 0.5–1 mg salt tds.
  - Further increases should follow according to response and tolerability. Maximum total daily dose is 4.5 mg salt daily.
- Oral long-lasting pramipexole once daily. Tablets provided: 0.375 mg salt (0.26 mg base), 0.75 mg salt (0.52 mg base), 1.5 mg salt (1.05 mg base), up to 4.5 mg salt (3.15 mg base).
  - Starting dose 0.375 mg salt (0.26 mg base), increasing every 5–7 days. Typical maintenance dose is 1.5–3 mg salt once daily.

*Ropinirole*
- A non-ergot agonist with affinity for D2 and D3 receptors.
- Tablets provided: 0.25 mg (white), 0.5 mg (yellow), 1 mg (green), 2 mg (pink), 5 mg (blue).
- Initiation is easiest with a 'starter pack' which titrates the patient with 0.25 and 0.5 mg tablets to 1 mg tds over 1 month, and a 'follow-on pack' which titrates the patient from 1 mg tds to 3 mg tds over a month.
- Typical initial maintenance dose is 3–5 mg tds. Maximum total daily dose is 24 mg.
- Long-lasting ropinirole to apply once daily 2–24 mg, starting with 2 mg and increasing by 2 mg every 2 weeks. Typical maintenance dose is 8–14 mg once daily.

*Rotigotine*
- A non-ergot agonist with affinity for D1, D2, and D3 receptors.
- Available as a skin patch which is changed every 24 hours.
- Patches provided are 2 mg/24 hours, 4 mg/24 hours, 6 mg/24 hours, and 8 mg/24 hours.
- Note that, in clinical trials of rotigotine, the doses stated are the actual amount of rotigotine in each patch, rather than the amount delivered to the patient/24 hours that is used for the licensed product. Therefore, the actual patches of 2, 4, 6, and 8 mg/24 hours contain 4.5 mg, 9 mg, 13.5 mg, and 18 mg of rotigotine, respectively.
- Patients should start with a 2 mg patch, replaced each day at approximately the same time.

- The dose should be increased every 1–2 weeks in 2 mg increments. Currently licensed maximum dose is 8 mg/24 hours as *de novo* therapy, and 16 mg/24 hours for adjuvant use.
- The site of application should be changed each day. Commonly used sites include the upper arms, thighs, and abdomen.
- Some patients develop patch application site reactions, leading to discontinuation in 3–5% of patients.

*Piribedil (not available in the UK)*
- A non-ergot agonist with relative selective affinity for D2 and D3 receptors.
- Available as 50 mg tablets; start with 50 mg once daily, and increase every 2 weeks by 50 mg to reach 50 mg tds. Usual maintenance dose is 150–250 mg a day, no higher than 300 mg/day.
- Available as prolonged-release tablets to be taken once daily, starting with 50 mg and increasing usually up to 150 mg.

*Apomorphine*
- An injectable dopamine agonist used in advanced PD and discussed in detail on ➔ p. 82.

## Switching dopamine agonists

In general, if a patient has failed to gain significant benefit from one dopamine agonist, then it is unlikely that another will be successful. However, there are circumstances in which it may be necessary to switch dopamine agonists. Recently, this has occurred when patients on ergot dopamine agonists have been switched to non-ergot agonists because of concerns about fibrotic reactions.

Table 3.3 gives a list of approximately equivalent doses of different dopamine agonists which can be helpful in selecting the correct dose when switching.

**Table 3.3** Approximate equivalent doses of dopamine agonists

| Bromocriptine | 2.5 mg tds | 10 mg tds | 15 mg tds |
|---|---|---|---|
| Pergolide | 0.25 mg tds | 1 mg tds | 1.5 mg tds |
| Rotigotine | 4 mg/daily | 12 mg/daily | 16 mg/daily |
| Ropinirole | 1 mg tds | 5 mg tds | 8 mg tds |
|  | (3 mg once daily) | (15 mg once daily) | (24 mg once daily) |
| Pramipexole | 0.25 mg tds | 1 mg tds | 1.5 mg tds |
|  | (0.75 mg once daily) | (3 mg once daily) | (4.5 mg once daily) |

# Monoamine oxidase inhibitors

Selegiline and rasagiline are monoamine oxidase B (MAO-B) inhibitors which prevent the breakdown of dopamine in the synapse. They are indicated for monotherapy and as adjunctive therapy in PD.

### Selegiline

- Available as generic tablets or as Eldepryl® in 5 mg and 10 mg tablets. It is also available as a dissolvable buccal preparation (Zelapar®) in a dose of 1.25 mg (equivalent to 10 mg tablet).
- The standard dosage of selegiline is 10 mg taken in the morning, but some people start with 5 mg. Zelapar® is available in only one dose of 1.25 mg. The tablet is placed on the tongue and allowed to dissolve. Patients should not drink or wash their mouth out for 5 minutes after taking Zelapar®.
- Side effects: selegiline hydrochloride is metabolized to amphetamine derivatives and therefore tends to have an alerting effect. This may be beneficial but can result in insomnia, hallucinations, and rarely psychosis. Other side effects include dry mouth and hypotension. Selegiline should not be given to those with active gastric or duodenal ulceration.
- Zelapar® does not undergo first-pass metabolism to amphetamine derivatives and therefore may have less of an alerting effect and be less likely to cause confusion or hallucinations.
- If given at doses of more than 10 mg, selegiline loses its selectivity for MAO-B and can block MAO-A, an enzyme involved in the metabolism of tyramine-containing foods such as cheese, smoked meat, and red wine. Blockade of MAO-A leads to excessive plasma levels of tyramine, and a hypertensive crisis may result, especially if levodopa is also being given.
- If taken in conjunction with a selective serotonin reuptake inhibitor (SSRI), selegiline can very rarely cause a 'serotonergic crisis'. Patients become dyskinetic, confused, and hypertensive. Treatment is supportive, combined with withdrawal of selegiline and the SSRI.

### Rasagiline

Rasagiline is a newer MAO-B inhibitor which is licensed for monotherapy and adjunctive therapy in PD. It is not metabolized to amphetamine derivatives so may have a better side effect profile than selegiline.

- Available in tablets of 1 mg (the standard daily dose).
- Rasagiline should be initiated at 1 mg once daily.
- Main side effects include dry mouth, anorexia, depression, and headache. Rasagiline is metabolized by the liver; therefore, drugs that block liver enzymes, e.g. ciprofloxacin, can cause plasma levels to rise.
- As with selegiline, potentially blockade of monoamine oxidase A (MAO-A) by rasagiline could lead to a hypertensive crisis with tyramine-rich foods. However, in practice, no cases of this have occurred, and dietary advice is not necessary for patients.
- As with selegiline, combination of rasagiline and SSRIs can rarely lead to a 'serotonergic crisis'.
- One milligram of rasagiline costs almost ten times as much as 10 mg of selegiline.

# Catechol-*O*-methyltransferase inhibitors

Entacapone and tolcapone are catechol-*O*-methyltransferase (COMT) inhibitors. When a peripheral dopa decarboxylase inhibitor is given with levodopa (as in all levodopa preparations), COMT becomes the major metabolic enzyme involved in peripheral levodopa breakdown. Therefore, COMT inhibitors decrease peripheral levodopa metabolism, increasing plasma levodopa levels and prolonging the effect. Entacapone works purely peripherally. Tolcapone crosses the blood–brain barrier to some extent, and there is evidence from animal studies that it also blocks COMT in the central nervous system (CNS).

## Entacapone

Entacapone is only given with levodopa and is primarily indicated to prolong the effect of each levodopa dose, e.g. in patients who find that their symptoms return before the next dose of levodopa is due.

- Available in 200 mg brown/orange tablets.
- Also available with co-careldopa as Stalevo® (see under levodopa).
- Entacapone should be added to every other dose of levodopa initially, and then increased to every dose. Maximum dose is 2 g (ten tablets) daily.
- Main side effects are nausea, diarrhoea, and abdominal pain. Patients may experience an increase in dyskinesia, and the levodopa dose may need to be decreased. Entacapone turns the urine a harmless red/brown colour.
- Stalevo® can be used as a more convenient way to take levodopa and entacapone in a single tablet.

## Tolcapone

Tolcapone is only given with levodopa and has similar indications to entacapone. During the first 6 months of licensing, three deaths from acute fulminant liver failure were reported in patients taking tolcapone. The licence was temporarily withdrawn in the UK but has now been granted again. It is suggested that the drug only be given if another COMT inhibitor has failed to have effect, and only under specialist supervision.

- Available in 100 mg yellow tablets.
- Liver function must be tested before treatment: every 2 weeks for the first year, every 4 weeks for the next 6 months, and every 8 weeks thereafter. If the dose is increased, then testing every 2 weeks should resume. A rise in liver enzymes should lead to immediate withdrawal of tolcapone.
- Patients should be counselled about possible hepatic side effects and to be vigilant regarding possible symptoms of liver failure.
- Other side effects include nausea, diarrhoea, and an increase in dyskinesia. Urine colour often becomes darker.
- Tolcapone should be initiated at 100 mg tds, making sure that the first dose is taken with levodopa.
- Maximum dose is 600 mg daily.

# Amantadine and the anticholinergics

## Amantadine

Amantadine is a drug originally developed as an antiviral agent, but which has a symptomatic benefit in PD via a number of putative mechanisms, including dopamine and noradrenaline reuptake blockade, an amphetamine-like action releasing pre-synaptic monoamine stores, a mild anticholinergic effect, and antagonism of N-methyl-D-aspartic acid (NMDA) receptors.

Amantadine has a minor effect on bradykinesia, rigidity, and gait disturbance in PD. Its main indication is as an anti-dyskinetic drug in patients who have developed levodopa-induced dyskinesia.

- Available in 100 mg red/brown capsules.
- Initiate at 100 mg once daily, increasing, if necessary, to 100 mg bd or tds.
- Main side effects are nausea, leg swelling, leg rash (livedo reticularis), hallucinations, and confusion. Amantadine can lower seizure threshold.
- Some patients find that amantadine can act as a slight stimulant, and so a dose taken late in the day can lead to insomnia.

## Anticholinergics

Anticholinergic drugs can be used to treat tremor in PD. Confusion is a prominent side effect, particularly in older patients in whom they are best avoided. Slow titration is the key to help avoid side effects. Withdrawal should also be gradual if possible.

A number of anticholinergics are available: trihexyphenidyl, benzatropine, orphenadrine, and procyclidine. Efficacy and side effects are similar across preparations. In our practice, we most commonly use trihexyphenidyl.

- Trihexyphenidyl (previously benzhexol).
- Available as generic tablets 2 mg and 5 mg (white, scored), or in syrup (5 mg/5 mL).
- Starting dose is 1 mg daily. Increase by 1 mg every 4–7 days to reach 1 mg tds. Then increase by 1 mg every 4–7 days to reach 2–4 mg tds.
- If side effects occur, dose titration should be stopped and then re-attempted after 1–2 weeks.
- Dose to treat tremor is usually 2–4 mg tds.
- Common side effects: dry mouth, dry eyes, nausea, confusion, constipation, urinary retention.
- Important contraindications: closed-angle glaucoma, cognitive impairment, prostatism.

# Treatment initiation

No issue in PD is more vexed or mired in controversy than when to start treatment and with which drug to start. No consensus exists amongst movement disorder specialists, and good-quality objective experimental evidence is lacking. Add to this the claims and counterclaims of different pharmaceutical companies, and the practitioner is left in a very confused and unsatisfactory position. We have given some general guidance regarding our practice in this area, but our advice is for practitioners to judge the evidence for themselves and to keep a watchful eye on the results of upcoming clinical trials. The recent NICE guidelines on the management of PD provide an excellent summary of the clinical trial evidence and are available online at http://www.nice.org.gov. Since almost all pharmaceutical trials are of relatively short duration, it is important to consider also long-term natural history studies lasting 10, 15, or even 20 years, which show that the long-term outcome for patients is no different whether they were started on a levodopa preparation or a dopamine agonist.

## When to start treatment: neuroprotection and deconditioning

It is common practice to start medication only when the patient is functionally disabled by their symptoms. This makes common sense; there seems little point in giving patients medication which may have side effects unless they require it.

However, claims have been made that some drugs are neuroprotective or 'disease-modifying'. If these claims are true, then these drugs should be started as soon as the diagnosis of PD is made. Patients treated with ropinirole and pramipexole have shown less change in serial fluorodopa PET or DAT-SPECT scans, compared with patients treated with levodopa. However, the *clinical* benefit in these studies has favoured levodopa.

Patients treated with rasagiline have a marginally better score on a PD rating scale after 1 year of treatment than patients who delayed starting rasagiline for 6 months. On the basis of these studies, it has been argued that ropinirole, pramipexole, and rasagiline may be neuroprotective. However, there has been intense debate regarding these claims, and, if any effect is present, it is clearly rather small.

Even if neuroprotection is not offered by current medications, there are some who suggest that early treatment may prevent 'deconditioning'. It has been suggested that early treatment may slow down some of the pathological changes which occur in the basal ganglia circuitry because of denervation. Also early treatment might prevent the deconditioning of muscles which can occur with increasing immobility. Not surprisingly, patients who delay treatment tend to have worse quality of life scores, compared to others who start treatment earlier, until they themselves start effective symptomatic treatment.

Our view is that there is currently no robust evidence that absolutely supports early treatment before the patient is functionally disabled, but that clinical trials that are currently ongoing may help to inform this debate. We continue to initiate treatment when functional disability (as judged by the patient) is present. We actively encourage our patients that a range of effective treatments are available.

## Treatment initiation

Levodopa is recognized as the most effective drug for the treatment of motor symptoms in PD. However, the long-term consequences of levodopa treatment, in terms of dyskinesia and fluctuations, can be serious, and this has persuaded many practitioners to try to withhold levodopa for as long as possible.

*De novo* agonist monotherapy, by delaying the introduction of levodopa, delays levodopa-induced fluctuations and dyskinesia, but, when later on levodopa is needed, these develop, often with an accelerated latency, because by then the disease is more advanced. Ongoing studies are examining whether giving levodopa in a way that reduces large peaks and troughs can reduce or delay dyskinesia, as is the case in animal models of PD.

The choice of drug with which to initiate therapy still depends largely on the age of the patient. Although levodopa has long-term side effects, it is still the initial treatment of choice in older patients with PD. Dopamine agonists cause hallucinations in many older patients, which increase in frequency and severity with increasing age. Monoamine oxidase (MAO) inhibitors (particularly the newer formulations) have a relatively good side effect profile, but only a fairly weak clinical effect. There are no absolute rules, and medication choice should be a matter of discussion between patient and doctor.

Importantly, the treatment pendulum initially swung away from starting with levodopa to starting with agonists in younger patients, but the last few years have seen a swing away from agonists, because they are much more expensive, less effective, and much more frequently cause potentially catastrophic ICDs, especially in younger-onset patients.

In contrast, levodopa's bad reputation for causing severe motor fluctuations and dyskinesia, when used in high dosages to achieve maximum clinical effect, has been tempered by sensible prescribing, keeping the dose as low as possible, and the sequelae of fluctuations and dyskinesia, particularly in younger-onset patients, can now be very well managed with STN DBS.

- Most specialist–patient pairings currently initiate with levodopa in patients with moderate motor symptoms over 65–70 years.
- Some initiate with a dopamine agonist in patients with moderate motor symptoms under 65–70 years, without dementia, but increasingly some prefer to start with levodopa and keep the dosage as low as possible.
- Many initiate with an MAO-B inhibitor in patients of any age with mild motor symptoms.
- Some initiate with an anticholinergic in patients under 60–65 years where tremor is the predominant disabling symptom and in young-onset (<40 years) PD, particularly if dystonia is a prominent clinical feature.

## Treatment titration

Dose of medication should be gradually increased, until an *acceptable* level of symptom control has been reached. This does not equate to complete abolition of all symptoms—patients should be counselled that the aim of treatment is to provide *adequate* control over troublesome symptoms. Aiming for more than this tends to lead to unacceptable side effects.

# Treatment of non-motor symptoms

### Dementia
As discussed on ➔ p. 36, some patients with PD present with prominent dementia (DLB), whereas others develop dementia much later in the course of the disease (PDD). These are probably different ends of the same spectrum of cognitive impairment which occurs with PD and have the same underlying mechanism. Other patients with PD may develop dementia due to incidental Alzheimer's disease or cerebrovascular disease.

There is evidence to support the use of the cholinesterase inhibitors rivastigmine (licensed for this indication in the UK) and donepezil (not currently licensed) in PDD and DLB. Despite initial concerns, there is no evidence that either drug significantly worsens parkinsonian symptoms. These drugs can improve cognitive function and can also reduce hallucinations that are a common feature of DLB.

### Depression and apathy
There is controlled trial evidence to support the use of SSRIs (fluoxetine, citalopram, and nefazodone) in depression associated with PD. Dopaminergic treatment itself, perhaps particularly pramipexole, may also improve depression in PD. In clinical practice, many other antidepressant drugs are used, but, for most, trial evidence for their efficacy is lacking, although nortriptyline was efficacious in a double-blind trial. Note that use of MAO inhibitors, such as selegiline and rasagiline, with SSRIs is theoretically contraindicated (➔ p. 60).

### Hallucinations and psychosis
Hallucinations and psychosis in PD occur in two common scenarios.
- In patients with DLB or PDD: spontaneous hallucinations and psychosis, which may be worsened by dopaminergic drugs or systemic illness such as infection.
- In patients without DLB or PDD: hallucinations and psychosis due to dopaminergic drugs or systemic illness.

Management is as follows.
- Assess the patient, and, if necessary, seek a psychiatric opinion. Are the hallucinations mild? If so, no treatment may be necessary. If they are severe, is the patient safe in their current environment, or is additional support needed (including psychiatric admission)?
- Is there an intercurrent illness (e.g. infection, electrolyte disturbance)?
- Assess medications. Hallucinations and psychosis may be helped by reduction in medications.
- Medications should be reduced on a 'last in, first out' basis. Medications most likely to cause hallucinations or psychosis are, in descending order, anticholinergics, amantadine, dopamine agonists, MAO inhibitors, COMT inhibitors, and levodopa.

- In patients with DLB/PDD, rivastigmine often improves symptoms. Atypical DRBs may also be used, but olanzapine and risperidone may lead to severe worsening of parkinsonian symptoms, and quetiapine is barely efficacious. Clozapine has class 1 evidence from two double-blind trials to support its efficacy, but it requires blood monitoring because of the risk of causing neutropenia. Therefore, it is commonly used as a second-line treatment after other choices, currently usually quetiapine, have failed to control symptoms.
- If DLB/PDD is not suspected as the cause, treatment with an atypical DRB is more suitable than with cholinesterase inhibitors.

## Sleep disturbance

Sleep disturbance in PD is multifactorial, and therefore the underlying cause needs to be carefully considered. Daytime somnolence is the commonest complaint and may be due to the following.

- 'Off'-period dystonia/pain at night: consider long-acting levodopa or dopamine agonist at night, or extra levodopa doses taken during the night.
- Use of dopamine agonists: consider reduction in dose/alternative medication.
- Sleep apnoea: consider sleep study to investigate.
- RBD: consider clonazepam at night, or melatonin.
- PLMS: consider clonazepam at night.
- Urinary frequency causing frequent wakenings: see Urinary dysfunction under Autonomic symptoms.

There have been controlled trials of modafinil for daytime somnolence in PD, some of which have suggested benefit without significant side effects.

## Autonomic symptoms

### Drooling

There have been a number of trials of BT type A injection into salivary glands to treat drooling in PD. Injections are given into the parotid glands alone, or into the parotid and submandibular glands. Some studies use ultrasound guidance. Good results have been reported, with few side effects and benefit lasting 3–4 months. Anticholinergic drugs, including hyoscine patches, can also be used but can cause confusion.

### Erectile dysfunction

Sildenafil has controlled trial evidence to support its use in the treatment of erectile dysfunction in PD. The main side effect is postural hypotension, and assessment of the degree of postural blood pressure drop should be undertaken prior to treatment initiation.

### Urinary dysfunction

Urinary dysfunction in PD has a complex aetiology. Assessment by a urologist and urodynamic studies can be very helpful to determine the cause of the urinary dysfunction and the role of non-neurogenic factors such as prostatic hypertrophy. Anticholinergic drugs, such as oxybutynin or tolterodine, can be helpful in improving urinary frequency, but these may cause confusion in patients with PD. Trospium, an alternative, is thought not to cross the blood–brain barrier.

# Physiotherapy, occupational therapy, and speech therapy

## Physiotherapy
There are a number of physiotherapy interventions that have been used in patients with PD at different stages of the condition. A recent Cochrane Review and the recent NICE guidelines have found some trial evidence in support of physiotherapy intervention in PD, but, at present, the best types of intervention are not well defined. The NICE guidelines suggest the following:
- gait re-education, improvement of balance and flexibility
- enhancement of aerobic capacity
- improvement of movement initiation
- improvement of functional independence, including mobility and activities of daily living
- provision of advice regarding safety in the home environment.

A large randomized controlled is currently under way in The Netherlands comparing 'routine' physiotherapy with a structured physiotherapy programme designed for people with PD. A detailed set of guidelines in Dutch and English and the specific aspects of the programme are available at http://www.kngf.nl.

## Occupational therapy
Very little trial evidence is available regarding the need for, and cost-effectiveness of, occupational therapy in PD. However, the provision of aids, the adjustment of the home environment, and the provision of advice and support regarding employment, where appropriate, are a valuable addition to the care of patients with PD. Further research into the cost-effectiveness of various occupational therapy strategies is needed.

## Speech and language therapy
Patients with PD frequently develop a progressively quiet, indistinct, and sometimes eventually unintelligible voice. There is controlled trial evidence to suggest that SLT can improve the volume and intelligibility of speech in patients with PD. In addition, speech and language therapists are experts in providing communication aids to patients whose speech cannot be improved.

Lee Silverman Voice Treatment (LSVT) is a specific speech therapy programme designed for patients with PD (http://www.lsvt.org). Developed in North America, it focuses mainly on improving the volume of speech. There are controlled studies supporting the efficacy of LSVT in PD, and it is suggested that this technique is more effective than standard SLT. However, LSVT is an intensive programme (16 1-hour sessions), and availability is limited in the UK. It is clear that SLT generally improves intelligibility of speech in people with PD and is a useful intervention in appropriate patients.

*Dysphagia*
Dysphagia is a problem which commonly develops in the later stages of PD and may lead to aspiration pneumonia. Patients may complain of coughing during eating or drinking, or frequent chest infections. Such patients should be seen urgently by speech and language therapists for a full assessment of their swallow (e.g. using video fluoroscopy) which will allow the appropriate dietary changes, or even gastrostomy feeding to be instituted if the patient wishes.

# Follow-up of patients with Parkinson's disease

Regular follow-up of patients with PD is important to review the diagnosis, evaluate symptom control, assess any complications of treatment, and look for the development of new symptoms (e.g. cognitive decline) which may require treatment.

## Documenting effectiveness of treatment

As PD progresses and the medication regime becomes more complex, it can be very difficult to gain a clear impression of the effectiveness or otherwise of medications. In such patients, it can be very helpful to draw a timeline for a typical 24-hour period, noting when each medication is taken and what the patient's symptoms are at each time point. In order for this to work, patients need to understand what is meant by being 'on' (free from troublesome symptoms of PD) and 'off' (troublesome symptoms of PD are present). It is also important for the patient to be able to indicate the occurrence of any dyskinesia. Fig. 3.2 is an example graph showing 24 hours in the life of a patient with PD.

## Important questions for the follow-up visit

- Review the diagnosis: is the diagnosis of PD secure?
- What medications are being taken and at what times? Draw along the *x* axis of the graph.
- What are the symptoms the patient experiences during the day (on, on with dyskinesia, off)? Pay particular attention to the response of symptoms to each dose of medication. Add these responses to the graph.
- What is the patient's impression of current symptom control?
- What side effects is the patient experiencing?
- Consider the need for a change in treatment for motor symptoms.
- Ask specifically about:
  - mood
  - cognition
  - hallucinations
  - change in behaviour (consider hypersexuality, paranoia, gambling)
  - daytime somnolence (if significant, advise to stop driving)
  - urinary symptoms
  - falls/gait disturbance
  - swallowing/speech.
- Consider the need for change in treatment/treatment initiation for non-motor symptoms.
- Consider the need for therapy referrals: physiotherapy, speech therapy, occupational therapy.
- Ask about social support: is there a need for additional help at home?
- Is the patient aware of/in touch with PDNS service, local PD patients association?
- Negotiate a follow-up visit.

FOLLOW-UP OF PATIENTS WITH PARKINSON'S DISEASE

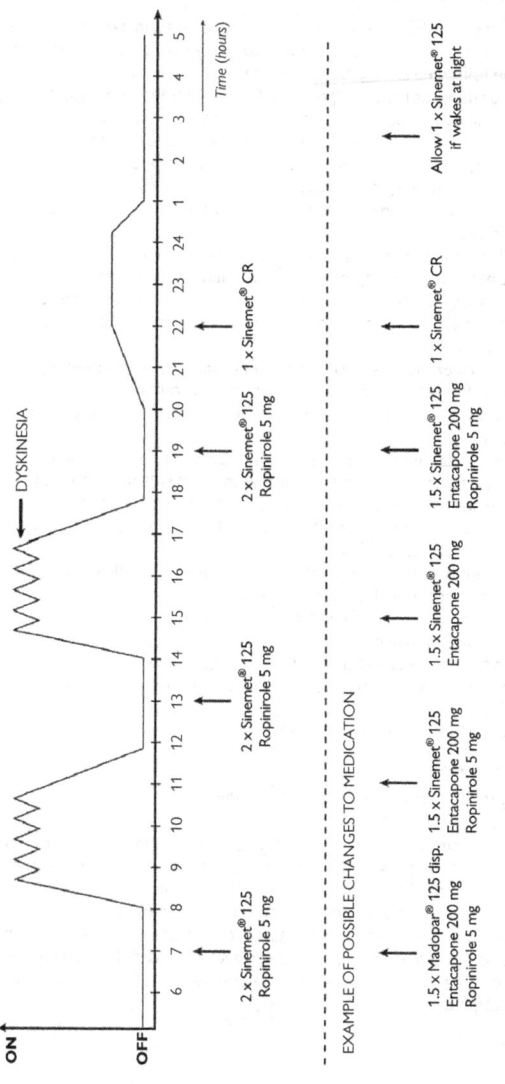

**Fig. 3.2** Timeline drawn at the follow-up of a typical patient with PD, with suggestions of how the medication might be changed to manage the clinical problems.

# Treatment escalation

Most patients with PD will notice a gradual increase in symptoms over time despite treatment. Before medication is increased in dose or altered, the following should be considered.

- What are the symptoms responsible for the patient's perception that PD has worsened? Non-motor symptoms, in particular depression, sleep disturbance, or urinary dysfunction, may be the main cause of worsening, which will not be helped by simply increasing dopaminergic medication.
- Ask the patient to prioritize the symptoms that they find most troublesome.
- Do not feel you have to try to address all of these at one visit—sometimes treating one symptom may worsen another.
- Try to only change one treatment parameter at a time, so that the result (beneficial or otherwise) can be correctly ascribed to the change made.
- Are there other factors unrelated to PD that may be worsening symptoms? PD tends to affect older people, who may have general medical problems, in addition to PD, which may be responsible for symptoms.
- Is the patient taking PD medication as directed? Patients should be encouraged to bring their medication with them to the outpatient clinic to ensure that the correct medication is being taken at the correct dose. Has the patient been prescribed any medication that may worsen PD (e.g. DRBs)?
- Is the patient having any side effects from current medication? These side effects may be the main cause of worsening symptoms and require an entirely different management from patients with worsening parkinsonism.
- Is the diagnosis of PD secure? Some patients with atypical parkinsonism have an initial response to dopaminergic drugs which is short-lived.
- What is the functional impact of the increase in symptoms?

## Common scenarios

*An unacceptable return of parkinsonian symptoms in patients on monotherapy*

This is a very common scenario which occurs some time after initiation of treatment with a dopamine agonist or levodopa. After consideration of the questions on ➔ p. 74, and if the patient is not experiencing side effects from current medication, in patients on dopamine agonists, the dose should be slowly increased until an acceptable level of symptom control has been achieved. In patients on levodopa, addition of a COMT inhibitor or dopamine agonist should be considered before an increase in the levodopa dose.

## TREATMENT ESCALATION

*An unacceptable level of parkinsonian symptoms in patients on maximum doses of dopamine agonists*

Despite dose increases, almost all patients on dopamine agonists will eventually experience the return of unacceptable parkinsonian symptoms. Switching dopamine agonists is rarely of benefit, and the addition of another dopamine agonist is not recommended. The main question with such patients is whether levodopa or another medication should be added. In younger patients (<60 years), a trial of an MAO-B inhibitor, in addition to the agonist, may be worthwhile before adding levodopa. In older patients, the addition of levodopa is usually the next step. The agonist can be continued after the addition of levodopa, but at a lower dose.

*Fluctuations in symptom control throughout the day*

Patients on long-term levodopa therapy often develop fluctuations in response to medication. These take various forms.
- **Early wearing off.** Patients experience a good response to each dose of medication, but a return of symptoms before their next dose of medication is due.
- **Slow time to on.** Patients experience a delay in response to a dose of medication.
- **Dose failure.** Despite taking a dose of medication, no appreciable response of motor symptoms is experienced.
- **Sudden off periods.** Without warning, the effect of medication suddenly completely disappears.

The management of these problems is greatly assisted by drawing a graph of a typical day for the patient, as described on ➲ p. 73. This provides a clear picture of medication response in relation to timings of doses. Where response is very variable, a diary (on–off chart) completed by the patient over a few days can be very helpful. Some strategies for dealing with these complications are as follows.
- **Early wearing off**: move doses of medication closer together; add a COMT inhibitor and/or an MAO-B inhibitor and/or a dopamine agonist.
- **Slow time to on**: increase dose; give medication in dispersible form; avoid high-protein meals prior to medication; add COMT/MAO-B inhibitor; stop anticholinergics.
- **Dose failure**: increase dose; try dispersible form; avoid high-protein meals prior to medication; consider apomorphine.
- **Sudden off periods**: move doses of medication closer together; give dispersible levodopa as 'rescue' therapy for sudden off periods; consider intermittent apomorphine injections as 'rescue' therapy.

*Development of gait disturbance/freezing*

This is a complex management problem. Gait disturbance and falls are multifactorial, and causes, such as postural hypotension, sedative drug use, and poor home environment, should be considered. Are the falls due to freezing or postural instability? The main categories of gait disturbance due to PD are as follows.

- **Off-period gait disturbance.** Patients have falls when they are 'off', but gait is well preserved when they are on. Such patients usually benefit from an increase in medication in order to create more 'on time' during the day. Off-period gait disturbance is not a contraindication to DBS surgery (➔ p. 86). Freezing may show some benefit with amantadine.
- **On-period gait disturbance.** Patients have falls whether they are on or off. This is much more problematic to treat and is usually a late feature of PD. Amantadine is sometimes of use. In a few patients, it is helped by reducing or gradually stopping a dopamine agonist. Occupational therapy and physiotherapy assessment are helpful, and provision of an adequate walking aid/wheelchair is essential. This type of gait disturbance is generally not improved by DBS surgery and additional poor balance contraindicates DBS. (➔ p. 86).
- **Gait disturbance due to dyskinesia.** Some patients with severe dyskinesia can be thrown off balance by the severity of the dyskinesia. Management of dyskinesia is discussed on ➔ p. 68.

TREATMENT ESCALATION

# Management of dyskinesias

Dyskinesias are involuntary choreiform or dystonic movements which occur following long-term treatment with levodopa in PD. Many patients have dyskinesias that are not troublesome, and, in these cases, no particular action is needed. However, troublesome dyskinesia is very difficult to treat, and a combination of approaches may be required (see Video 3.3: Levodopa-induced dyskinesia).

## Preventing dyskinesias

Dyskinesias are clearly related to the pulsatile nature of levodopa therapy. In the normal basal ganglia, there is a constant low-level activity at dopaminergic synapses, with transient increases during particular tasks such as voluntary movement and learning. With levodopa therapy in PD, this is replaced with large variations in the levels of dopamine, which result in abnormal patterns of basal ganglia activity in some patients, producing dyskinesias.

- Factors related to the risk of developing dyskinesias are:
  - longer duration of levodopa therapy
  - higher doses of levodopa
  - younger onset of PD.
- Dyskinesias may be delayed by ensuring that:
  - levodopa is only used if other treatments are of insufficient benefit or cause unacceptable side effects
  - levodopa dose is kept as low as possible through the use of other medications with levodopa such as COMT inhibitors, MAO-B inhibitors, and dopamine agonists, if side effects allow.
- The concept of continuous dopaminergic stimulation (CDS) has been proposed as a method of avoiding dyskinesia. In fact, rather than CDS, it appears that simply avoiding large peaks and troughs in dopaminergic stimulation is the most important. However, in studies, neither the addition of entacapone nor the use of long-acting preparations of levodopa have reduced the incidence of dyskinesias.
- A system for infusing levodopa–carbidopa directly into the jejunum through a gastrostomy tube is available (Duodopa®) (p. 84). This leads to more stable levodopa levels and therefore may increase on-time without worsening dyskinesias. However, the system requires an invasive procedure and is expensive.

## Types of dyskinesia

There are three main types of dyskinesia.

- **Peak-dose dyskinesia**: dyskinesias occur when levodopa levels are at their highest. Often they are much the same throughout the on period ('square-wave dyskinesias').
- **Off-period dyskinesia**: occurs when levodopa levels are at their lowest. Rather than choreiform movements, this often comprises relatively fixed and often painful abnormal postures (dystonia).

- **Biphasic dyskinesia**: dyskinesias occur when the levels of levodopa are rising, then reduce or disappear when levodopa levels are above a certain threshold, and finally return when levels fall again. Therefore, patients experience dyskinesias as the drug begins to take effect, and again when the effect begins to wear off ('beginning-and-end-of-dose dyskinesias').

## Treatment of dyskinesia

### Peak-dose dyskinesia
- If treatment is needed, the first step is to reduce the dose of levodopa. This should reduce the severity of dyskinesia but may lead to an unacceptable return of parkinsonian symptoms.
- Dopamine agonists or COMT inhibitors can allow the dose of levodopa to be reduced.
- Introduce amantadine (⊃ p. 64).
- Consider apomorphine (⊃ p. 82) or DBS (⊃ p. 86).

### End-of-dose dystonia
- If symptoms are only occurring at night (e.g. patients may be woken in the early hours of the morning by a painful abnormal posture of the foot), consider giving long-acting preparations of levodopa, or a dopamine agonist just before bedtime. Alternatively, patients could take a tablet of dispersible levodopa if they wake with dystonia during the night.
- If symptoms are occurring during the day, doses of levodopa can be moved closer together.
- A COMT inhibitor can be added to each dose of levodopa.
- Consider apomorphine (⊃ p. 82).

### Biphasic dyskinesias
- A common error is to misdiagnose biphasic dyskinesia as peak-dose dyskinesia and reduce the dose of medication. This tends to place patients at the plasma level of levodopa that causes dyskinesia for a longer period of time, therefore worsening their symptoms.
- The main aim of treatment of biphasic dyskinesias is to try to keep the plasma level of levodopa above that which causes dyskinesias.
- Individual doses of levodopa may need to be increased and/or moved further apart to give predictable complete on–off cycles.
- Long-acting levodopa preparations may worsen these dyskinesias, necessitating a switch back to standard preparations.
- Try amantadine (⊃ p. 64).
- Consider apomorphine (⊃ p. 82).
- Consider DBS (⊃ p. 86).

# Non-motor side effects of dopaminergic therapy

Dyskinesias and fluctuations in response to treatment are the commonest motor complications of dopaminergic therapy. However, a number of non-motor side effects may also occur.

## Neuropsychiatric side effects
- Hallucinations and psychosis (● p. 68).
- Hypersexuality: this is more commonly reported with dopamine agonists than with other dopaminergic drugs. Symptoms range from a simple increase in libido to inappropriate, and sometimes aggressive, sexually motivated behaviour. Also, morbid jealousy can occur.
- Pathological gambling: this is more commonly associated with dopamine agonists than with other dopaminergic drugs.

### The dopamine dysregulation syndrome
Some patients treated with dopaminergic drugs develop a pattern of behaviour where they take ever increasing doses of medication. Such patients are often very dyskinetic but, despite this, will insist on the need for more medication. Patients may display features of 'addiction' to dopaminergic drugs, e.g. hoarding medication, lying to medical professionals and their carers about their medication intake, and an intense fear of being without medication.

This behaviour is most commonly seen in patients treated with levodopa. Treatment as an outpatient may be very difficult, and admission (often to a psychiatric ward) may be needed. Gradual reduction in medication dose should be negotiated with the patient, together with an exploration of the reasons for over-medication. A suitable regimen of treatment should be agreed. The patient's general practitioner (GP) should be informed of the issues regarding medication overuse and of the need to ensure that any increases in medication dose are discussed in advance with the neurologist. With the patient's consent, it can be helpful to visit their home to ensure that no supplies of medication have been hoarded.

Punding is a type of behaviour first described in chronic users of amphetamines, which is also sometimes seen in people with dopamine dysregulation syndrome. It consists of repetitive meaningless activity, often carried out for days on end, at the expense of all other activities (e.g. disassembling household objects, sorting papers or coins).

## Sleep disturbance
Dopaminergic drugs can impair sleep in two main ways.
- Daytime somnolence: commonly reported with dopamine agonists, but also occurs with levodopa. Sudden onset of sleep, or 'sleep attack', is a recognized complication of dopamine agonist therapy, and patients should be counselled regarding this. Patients with daytime somnolence and sleep attacks should stop driving.
- Insomnia: amantadine and MAO-B inhibitors can cause insomnia and should not be taken in the evening. Large doses of levodopa can also cause insomnia.

# Apomorphine

Apomorphine is one of the oldest synthesized drugs still in general use. It was discovered in 1869 when it was found that dehydration of morphine produced a new compound. Apomorphine is a dopamine agonist that is solely used in an injectable form. Treatment with apomorphine requires specialist supervision, usually with a dedicated service led by a PDNS, in close liaison with local GPs and district nurses. Apomorphine can be a very useful adjunct to therapy, particularly in those with advanced disease or levodopa-related complications.

## Indications for apomorphine

- On–off fluctuations not responsive to other measures (➲ p. 75).
- Peak-dose, end-of-dose, or biphasic dyskinesia not responsive to other measures (➲ p. 78).
- Inadequate response of motor symptoms to current therapy, despite medication changes.

## Methods of administration

### Single injections

Apomorphine can be given as a single subcutaneous injection. The main indication for this method of administration is sudden off periods occurring fewer than six times per day. Patients (or their caregivers) can give an injection subcutaneously, and a beneficial response usually occurs within minutes. Apomorphine for this purpose is available in a 'pen' device, pre-filled with 30 mg of apomorphine, or as a vial of apomorphine which can be drawn up into a syringe.

### Continuous subcutaneous infusion

Apomorphine can be given via an external pump connected to the patient though a needle placed subcutaneously. A pre-filled syringe containing 50 mg of apomorphine is attached to the pump. The main indications for this method of administration are inadequate response to other therapy, sudden off periods occurring more than six times per day, and sometimes end-of-dose dyskinesia/dystonia.

## Starting apomorphine

### Single injections

- Pretreat patients with domperidone 20 mg tds for 3 days.
- Ideally, admit the patient for an overnight stay, and do not give morning medications. Assess the patient at baseline, using the same methods as the levodopa challenge (➲ p. 41).
- Give increasing doses of apomorphine (1.5 mg, 3 mg, 4.5 mg, 7 mg) every 45 minutes, assessing response as at baseline 20 minutes after each dose. Once there is a >20% improvement in Unified Parkinson's Disease Rating (UPDRS) or timed tests of hand movement or walking, no further doses are given.
- Restart the patient on normal medication, and advise to use half the effective dose identified in the apomorphine test as treatment for sudden off periods, increasing the dose if there is no or inadequate response.

*Continuous infusion*
- Perform assessments, as described for the apomorphine test, to identify whether the patient responds to apomorphine and the dose at which response occurs.
- Patients usually require admission for several days in order to initiate and begin titrating the dose of apomorphine, and to modify other medications.
- Initiate the pump at 0.2 mL/hour, and monitor the response.
- Dopamine agonists should be stopped or tailed off. The dose of levodopa should be reduced, usually by about 30–50% initially. Sometimes, it may be possible to stop levodopa altogether, but most patients will continue to need some.
- Pump rate should be increased in 0.2 mL/hour increments every day, until a suitable dose is found.
- The subcutaneous needle can be placed on the abdomen below the umbilicus and on the anterior thigh.
- The dose of apomorphine (in mg) being delivered to the patient is five times that of the flow rate of the pump. Therefore, a flow rate of 0.2 mL/hour gives an apomorphine dose of 1 mg/hour.

## Side effects of apomorphine
- Nausea or vomiting are common but can be treated using domperidone, and tolerance usually develops.
- Other side effects include hallucinations, psychosis, hypersexuality, sleep disturbance, dyskinesia, penile erection, yawning, and sedation.
- Subcutaneous nodules often form at injection sites. These may be painful and can become infected. Rotation of injection sites is essential, and an aseptic technique is important when inserting the needle. Gentle massage of the injection sites can also help prevent nodule formation.
- Haemolytic anaemia is a rare complication of apomorphine infusion, and periodic assessment of full blood count and a Coombs test are recommended.

# Duodopa®

Duodopa® is an intestinal gel formulation of levodopa and carbidopa for continuous duodenal application. Continuous administration of dopaminergic agents via a non-oral route avoids fluctuations in absorption that are due to delayed gastric emptying and diet-related competition for intestinal uptake mechanisms. Duodopa® treatment needs close monitoring, in particular due to technical problems that can frequently occur in relation to the gastrostomy or infusion system.

### Indications for Duodopa®
- Duodopa® is indicated in patients with advanced PD with severe motor fluctuations when available combinations of current Parkinson's medications are unsatisfactory.
- Usually it offers an alternative to patients with advanced PD who are not suitable candidates for DBS, due to advanced age or psychiatric and cognitive dysfunction.
- A positive response to a nasogastric infusion is required before inserting the gastrostomy.

### Administration
- Usually a percutaneous endoscopic gastroscopy (PEG) is performed.
- Duodopa® is available in gel containing 20 mg levodopa/5 mg carbidopa.
- Usually there is a morning bolus dose, a maintenance dose, as well as an extra bolus, if needed.

### Side effects of Duodopa® pump
- The commonest reported problems are technical and related to the gastrostomy with dislocations or disconnections of the tube, or surgical complications with infections or inflammation.
- Polyneuropathy related to the drug itself.
- Hallucinations, psychosis, or worsening of dyskinesias, which usually improve with adjustments of the dose and oral drugs.

# Deep brain stimulation

Neurosurgery for PD has a long history, particularly lesion operations on the thalamus to treat tremor and on the pallidum to treat dyskinesia. DBS of the STN has largely replaced these lesion operations and offers significant benefit to carefully selected patients with PD.

### Technical aspects of deep brain stimulation

DBS involves the insertion through a small craniotomy of small-diameter electrodes into the selected target. The electrode leads are then tunnelled under the skin and connected to electrical pulse generators implanted underneath the skin, usually in the upper chest. Electrodes are inserted using stereotactic guidance where a metal frame is placed on the patient's head, and an MRI scan is performed. The position of the target is then referred to the metal frame, and a computer is used which enables planning of the correct track along which the electrodes should be inserted. Intraoperative micro-electrode recordings may be used to ensure correct placement, and macro-electrode stimulation to determine the therapeutic range between clinically effective stimulation parameters and the development of off-target side effects.

Intraoperative MRI guidance without micro-electrode recordings, provides the benefit of being able to use general anesthesia, and is being increasingly adopted utilising either frame-based or frameless techniques.

### Timing of the surgery

Traditionally, DBS surgery has been performed in patients with advanced PD. Recently, the effects of DBS in younger patients (<60 years) with early disease stage (Hoehn and Yahr stage <3) has been proven of benefit.

### Patient selection for deep brain stimulation

Correct patient selection is essential for the success of DBS. In general, DBS will provide patients with as good a response as they get to medication, but without dyskinesia or fluctuations. Symptoms that do not respond to medication will not usually be improved by DBS. Main criteria for selection are as follows:
- good response to levodopa, but at the expense of dyskinesias and/or fluctuations that cannot be managed using other methods
- no on-period freezing of gait or significant postural instability
- no significant dementia
- no significant psychiatric disturbance
- age under 70 (although higher age is not an absolute contraindication).

Patients put forward for DBS are usually assessed by a specialist neurosurgical/neurological team with brain imaging, neuropsychometry, psychiatric assessment, and a levodopa challenge test.

### Target selection for deep brain stimulation

The commonest targets are currently the STN and GPi. The GPi was the first target used for PD, but, since the introduction of STN DBS, the latter is now more often the target. Although STN DBS seems to cause more frequently psychiatric and neurocognitive side effects, to date, these two targets are considered equally effective in treating the major motor symptoms of PD. The STN is usually used in patients with severe off periods, while the GPi may be considered more often in patients with severe dyskinesias. New targets, such as the pedunculopontine nucleus (PPN) for treating postural instability, the nucleus basalis of Meynert for treating neurocognitive symptoms, or a combination of several targets, are currently under investigation.

### Possible side effects of deep brain stimulation

- Brain haemorrhage.
- Worsening of psychiatric/cognitive disturbance.
- Speech disturbance.
- Lead infection, fracture.

### Follow-up after deep brain stimulation

Following DBS, patients typically stay in hospital for recovery and commencement of stimulation. Stimulator settings (intensity of stimulation, pulse frequency) are adjusted according to response. Ideally, medications are gradually reduced, as the stimulator begins to work. Regular assessment is required, especially in the first few months after stimulator insertion, to adjust stimulator settings.

# The Parkinson's disease nurse specialist

A network of PDNS is well established within the UK and forms part of best practice in the care of patients with PD. The recent NICE report on the management of PD (→ p. 49) proposes that a number of the recommendations of the report could be delivered by a PDNS. The possible responsibilities of the PDNS include the following:

- follow-up of patients with an established diagnosis in the outpatient clinic, via home visit, or by telephone consultation. This follow-up could include assessment of symptom control, adjustment in current medication, and initiation of new medication
- allowing rapid access to telephone advice regarding PD symptoms and treatment for patients and carers
- assessment of inpatients with PD or suspected PD as part of the neurology inpatient service
- administering apomorphine challenges/initiation of apomorphine treatment within the hospital
- management of outpatient apomorphine service
- assisting in the assessment of patients referred for DBS surgery
- facilitation and coordination of referral to other services (e.g. occupational therapy, physiotherapy, SLT, social services, palliative care)
- facilitating communication between patient and consultant neurologist (e.g. need for more urgent outpatient review, information on response to newly initiated therapy)
- education of therapists, doctors, students, and primary care workers regarding PD and its management
- education of patients and carers regarding PD
- audit of PD management within the hospital or primary care setting
- participating in research regarding PD and its management.

The degree to which PDNS can adjust or initiate drug treatments for patients depends on local policies. The current NHS push towards the establishment of 'nurse consultant' posts is likely to extend the ability of PDNS to alter and prescribe medication. Although studies have not found PDNS to reduce costs associated with the management of patients with PD, they do improve the quality of life and level of care for PD patients. As well as delivering care and education themselves, PDNS provide a vital bridge between the patient and health and social services.

For further information regarding the PDNS network in the UK, visit http://www.pdnsa.org/.

# Measuring Parkinson's disease severity

## Hoehn and Yahr staging

In 1967, Hoehn and Yahr published the results of a long-term follow-up study of 204 patients with PD, documenting how long it took for patients to reach each stage of a 5-point symptom scale. This scale has continued to be used but has now been modified to include scores of 1.5 and 2.5. It was a descriptive scale to describe stages of PD progression and was never designed to document improvement, as it pre-dated the discovery of effective treatment for PD.

- **Stage 1**: symptoms on one side of the body only
- **Stage 1.5**: symptoms on one side of the body and axial symptoms
- **Stage 2**: symptoms on both sides of the body; no impairment of balance
- **Stage 2.5**: symptoms on both sides of the body plus recovery on the pull test
- **Stage 3**: balance impairment; mild to moderate disease; physically independent
- **Stage 4**: severe disability, but still able to walk or stand unassisted
- **Stage 5**: wheelchair-bound or bedridden unless assisted

## MDS Unified Parkinson's Disease Rating Scale[1]

This is the most widely used scale to assess patients with PD. It consists of four sections. In practice, only the third section (the motor scale) is generally used.

- Section I: mentation, behaviour, mood
- Section II: activities of daily living
- Section III: motor examination
- Section IV: complications of therapy

The maximum score is 199, indicating the worst possible clinical state. A score of zero indicates no symptoms.

## Other scales

The above scales clearly place the emphasis on motor symptoms and do not fully capture the range of disability caused by PD. Other scales are commonly used in conjunction with the UPDRS in order to measure these aspects of PD and include the Schwab and England Activities of Daily Living Scale and SF-36, a quality of life scale. A scale specifically focusing on non-motor symptoms in PD has also recently been developed[2].

---

1 Goetz CG1, Tilley BC, Shaftman SR, et al. Movement Disorder Society-sponsored revision of the Unified Parkinson's Disease Rating Scale (MDS-UPDRS): scale presentation and clinimetric testing results. Mov Disord. 2008 Nov 15;23(15):2129–70.

2 Chaudhuri KR, Martinez-Martin P, Schapira AH, et al. (2006). International multicenter pilot study of the first comprehensive self-completed nonmotor symptoms questionnaire for Parkinson's disease: the NMSQuest study. *Mov Disord*, **21**(7), 916–23

# Useful websites and addresses

- **Parkinsons UK**: 216 Vauxhall Bridge Road, London, SW1V 1EJ. Tel: 020 7931 8080; http://www.parkinsons.org.uk. National helpline: 0808 800 0303. National PD society. Has a network of local branches and also a young-onset PD group within the organization.
- **European Parkinson's Disease Association (EPDA)**: 1 Cobden Road, Sevenoaks, Kent, TN13 3UB. http://www.epda.eu.com/en/PD association linking PD associations in 38 European countries.
- **American Parkinson Disease Association**: 135 Parkinson Avenue, Staten Island, NY 10305; http://www.apdaparkinson.org.
- **National Parkinson Foundation (USA)**: 200 SE 1st Street, Suite 800, Miami, FL 33131; http://www.parkinson.org.
- **Michael J Fox Foundation for Parkinson's Research (USA)**: Grand Central Station, PO Box 4777, New York, NY 10163-4777; http://www.michaeljfox.org.
- **Parkinson's Disease Specialist Nurse Association (UK)**: http://www.pdnsa.org/.
- **International Parkinson and Movement Disorder Society**: formerly MDS (Movement Disorder Society); http://www.movementdisorders.org. International society for all movement disorders, including PD.

# Chapter 4

# Atypical parkinsonism

Introduction *94*
Progressive supranuclear palsy *96*
Imaging in progressive supranuclear palsy *100*
Multiple system atrophy *102*
Imaging in multiple system atrophy *106*
Corticobasal degeneration *108*
Differentiating Parkinson's disease, multiple system atrophy, progressive supranuclear palsy, and corticobasal degeneration *112*
Mechanisms of neurodegeneration *114*
Other degenerative causes of parkinsonism *116*
Secondary causes of parkinsonism *120*
Useful websites and addresses *122*

# Atypical parkinsonism

## Introduction

This chapter will cover 'atypical parkinsonism'—causes of parkinsonism, apart from PD. There are a number of degenerative causes of atypical parkinsonism, including PSP, MSA, and CBD. The main difficulty with these conditions is that they can easily be confused with PD, and there are almost no reliable diagnostic tests to tell them apart. Often the diagnosis will become clearer with time, as most of these atypical parkinsonian conditions respond poorly, if at all, to levodopa, are more rapidly progressive than PD, and have additional symptoms or signs not usually associated with PD (e.g. eye movement disorder, cerebellar signs). However, differentiation of the atypical conditions themselves is also very challenging (Table 4.1).

Table 4.1 Causes of parkinsonism

| | |
|---|---|
| Heredo-degenerative causes of parkinsonism | Parkinson's disease |
| | (Parkinson's disease—sporadic and genetic forms) |
| | Dementia with Lewy bodies (DLB) |
| | Progressive supranuclear palsy (PSP) |
| | Multiple system atrophy (MSA) |
| | Corticobasal degeneration (CBD) |
| | Alzheimer's disease (AD) |
| | Pick's disease |
| | Huntington's disease (HD) |
| | Parkinsonism–amyotrophic lateral sclerosis–dementia complex of Guam |
| | Fronto-temporal dementia with parkinsonism linked to chromosome 17 (FTDP-17) |
| | Lubag (X-linked dystonia parkinsonism); basal ganglia calcification (Fahr's syndrome); fragile X-associated tremor/ataxia syndrome (FXTAS) |
| | Dopa-responsive dystonia (DRD) |
| | Neuroacanthocytosis |
| | Dentatorubropallidoluysian atrophy (DRPLA) |
| | Neuronal brain iron accumulation syndromes (NBIAs) |
| | Spinocerebellar ataxias (esp. SCA 3) |
| | Pallidal degeneration syndromes (e.g. Kufor–Rakeb) |
| | Neuronal intranuclear inclusion disease |
| | Rapid-onset dystonia parkinsonism (RODP) |
| | Neurofilament inclusion body disease |
| Secondary causes of parkinsonism | Drugs (esp. dopamine receptor-blocking drugs) |
| | Toxins (e.g. manganese, MPTP), vascular disease |
| | Post-encephalitic (e.g. Japanese B encephalitis) |
| | Neurosyphilis |
| | Anoxic brain injury |
| | Traumatic brain injury (dementia pugilistica); basal ganglia lesions (esp. involving the substantia nigra) |
| | Metabolic disorders (e.g. Wilson's disease, GM1 gangliosidosis) |
| | Causes of basal ganglia calcification (e.g. hypoparathyroidism) |
| | Hydrocephalus |

# Progressive supranuclear palsy

PSP is a degenerative disease characterized by symmetrical parkinsonism, cognitive changes, a characteristic supranuclear (upper motor neuron) palsy of vertical gaze, early falls, dysarthria, and dysphagia.

## Historical aspects

The first recognized clinical description of PSP was given by J Richardson, an American neurologist, in 1963. The pathological features of the condition were described in the same year by the pathologist J Olszewski, and, in the following year, a fuller description of the syndrome was given in a paper written with J Steele. Following this publication, PSP became known as 'Steele–Richardson–Olszewski syndrome', although, in recent times, further changes in name have been suggested.

## Epidemiology

- Prevalence is approximately 5 per 100 000.
- Men and women are equally affected.
- Average age at onset is 63, and mean time from symptom onset to death is 7 years. No proven cases have begun before age 40. PSP is almost always sporadic, and only a handful of familial cases have been reported (see Genetics of progressive supranuclear palsy).

## Genetics of progressive supranuclear palsy

- The commonest risk allele for PSP is the H1 haplotype of the *MAPT* (microtubule-associated protein tau) gene.
- A genome-wide association study has identified further risk factors, including *EIF2AK3, STX6*, and *MOBP* genes, but their pathophysiological relevance is still unclear.
- Rarely, familial cases have been reported with mutations in the *MAPT* gene.

## Pathology

PSP is a 'tauopathy'—a disorder associated with abnormal aggregates of the tau protein ('4-repeat tau'). PSP is characterized pathologically by the degeneration of several subcortical structures, including the substantia nigra, STN, and midbrain. Neurofibrillary tangles are present in these areas. Tufted astrocytes (Gallyas-positive) are the hallmark feature of PSP that differentiates it in pathology from other 4R tauopathies such as CBD (astrocytic plaques).

## Clinical features

- Symmetrical parkinsonism, usually without tremor (see Video 4.1: PSP).
- Prominent neck dystonia, leading to stiffness and rarely to retrocollis.
- Markedly reduced blink rate.
- Closure of eyelids due to 'levator inhibition' (also known as 'apraxia of eyelid opening'), resulting in overactivity of the frontalis in an attempt to keep the eyelids open (surprised look).

- Slowed vertical saccades progressing (possibly over several years) to a vertical supranuclear gaze palsy (paresis). The doll's eye manoeuvre in PSP is normal. Note that many older people have a limitation of upgaze. This is not usually pathological, but a limitation of downgaze is always abnormal. In late-stage PSP, the eyes may become relatively fixed, and there may be little or no correction with the doll's eye manoeuvre.
- Postural instability leading to early falls (often backwards). Patients often display 'motor recklessness' where, despite frequent falls, they display no caution in the way that they walk, throwing themselves into and out of chairs, taking no account of their lack of balance.
- Dementia, often with frontal/executive dysfunction.
- Dysarthria and dysphagia.
- Lack of levodopa response (but see treatment of PSP).

### The doll's head manoeuvre and progressive supranuclear palsy

- Impairment of vertical saccades is the most striking feature in PSP, but vertical pursuit eye movements can also be impaired, so that the patient is unable to follow a target up or down.
- If there is limitation of vertical eye movements, the doll's head manoeuvre should be performed to check if the eye movement disorder is supranuclear.
- This manoeuvre assesses a brainstem reflex which is preserved until late in PSP.
- The patient is asked to fixate on a point straight ahead (usually the examiner's nose).
- The examiner then takes the patient's head in their hands and moves it up and down (quite difficult, as the neck can be very stiff in PSP).
- A normal (or near-normal) range of vertical eye movements will be seen in PSP. This demonstrates that the basic apparatus for moving the eyes up and down from the nucleus, down the nerve, and to the muscle is intact, and that the problem is above this, i.e. supranuclear.

*Clinical criteria for progressive supranuclear palsy diagnosis*
There are several sets of criteria proposed to diagnose PSP, but the most widely used are[1]: a progressive disorder with onset >40 years
- possible PSP: either vertical supranuclear gaze palsy, or slowing of vertical saccades and postural instability with falls within the first year
- probable PSP: vertical supranuclear gaze palsy and falls within the first year
- definite PSP: pathology required.

---

1 Litvan I, Agid Y, Calne D, *et al.* (1996). Clinical research criteria for the diagnosis of progressive supranuclear palsy (Steele-Richardson-Olszewski syndrome): report of the NINDS-SPSP international workshop. *Neurology*, 47(1), 1–9.

These criteria have shown high specificity but low sensitivity in diagnosing PSP. A particular problem is that many PSP patients do not fall during the first year, so they can only ever be possible cases until they come to autopsy when they become definite.

*Progressive supranuclear palsy phenotypes*
The 'typical' PSP phenotype is now termed Richardson's syndrome (RS), with an average survival of 6 years. The second commonest phenotype seems to be PSP-parkinsonism (PSP-P) resembling PD, with asymmetric parkinsonism, rest tremor, better levodopa response, and longer mean survival of 9 years. These together explain the mean PSP survival of 7 years. Further phenotypes include pure akinesia with gait freezing (PAGF), corticobasal syndrome (CBS), fronto-temporal dementia (FTD), progressive non-fluent aphasia (PNFA), and cerebellar ataxia (PSP-C). The relative frequency and natural distribution of these phenotypes are not known but may partly account for the low sensitivity of diagnosing PSP, based on current clinical criteria.

## Investigation of progressive supranuclear palsy

There are no diagnostic tests for PSP, and it remains a clinical diagnosis. Supportive features on investigation include the following.
- Absence of cardiovascular autonomic dysfunction (however, bladder disturbances are common).
- MRI findings of atrophy of superior cerebellar peduncles, midbrain atrophy, high signal in midbrain, atrophy or signal increase in the red nucleus, and signal increase in the globus pallidus (Fig. 4.1).
- Functional imaging: DAT scans are abnormal in MSA, PSP, and PD. To differentiate from PD, [$^{123}$I]meta-iodobenzylguanidine (MIBG) may be useful. MIBG is a tracer binding to cardiac sympathetic neurons and is abnormal in PD because of post-ganglionic sympathetic denervation, but is typically normal in PSP. Iodobenzamide (IBZM) SPECT assessing the post-synaptic receptors is abnormal in PSP, and normal in PD. However, MIBG scintigraphy cannot differentiate between PSP and other atypical parkinsonian conditions such as MSA or CBD.

## Treatment of progressive supranuclear palsy

- There is no treatment that alters the course of the disease.
- Supportive treatment, particularly regarding swallowing and prevention of falls, prolongs survival and improves quality of life.
- A trial of levodopa (up to 1 g/day) and amantadine is worthwhile.
- BT injections can be used to treat levator inhibition.

## Conditions confused with progressive supranuclear palsy: the PSP lookalike syndromes

| | |
|---|---|
| Sporadic neurodegenerative disorders (commonly) | Corticobasal degeneration<br>Fronto-temporal dementia<br>Parkinson's disease<br>Dementia with Lewy bodies<br>Multiple system atrophy<br>Alzheimer's disease<br>Cerebral amyloid angiopathy<br>Prion (rarely)<br>Motor neuron disease (rarely) |
| Vascular | Cerebrovascular disease<br>Thoracic aneurysm surgery (rarely)<br>CADASIL (rarely) |
| Infectious | Whipple disease<br>Neurosyphilis<br>Human immunodeficiency virus |
| Autoimmune/paraneoplastic | Ma2 encephalitis<br>Antiphospholipid syndrome<br>PERM (antiglycine antibodies)<br>Neurosarcoidosis |
| Genetic conditions | Genetic fronto-temporal dementia/amyotrophic lateral sclerosis overlap syndromes (*C9ORF72, MAPT, PRGN, FUS*)<br>Niemann–Pick type C, Gaucher's disease<br>Perry syndrome (*DCNT1* mutations) (rarely)<br>Leukoencephalopathy with spheroids (*CSF1R* mutations) |

## CHAPTER 4 Atypical parkinsonism

# Imaging in progressive supranuclear palsy

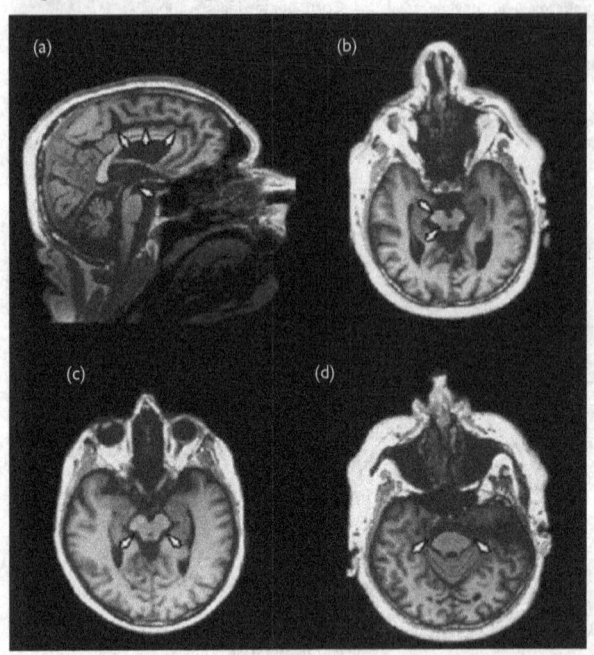

**Fig. 4.1** (a) Sagittal routine T1-weighted magnetic resonance images showing frontal lobe atrophy (three white arrows) and the 'hummingbird sign' (one arrow) in the sagittal plane. (b) The classical 'Mickey Mouse sign' indicating midbrain atrophy on axial slices. (c) The 'morning glory sign' with concavity of the lateral margin of the midbrain tegmentum also indicating midbrain atrophy on axial slices. (d) Atrophy of the superior cerebellar peduncle on axial slices.

Reproduced from J Neurol, 258(4), Stamelou M, Knake S, Oertel WH, Höglinger GU, Magnetic resonance imaging in progressive supranuclear palsy, pp. 549–58, Copyright (2011), with permission from Springer.

## Multiple system atrophy

MSA is a degenerative disorder characterized by parkinsonism, and/or cerebellar signs, and autonomic failure. The name multiple system atrophy was coined in 1969, unifying under one name Shy–Drager syndrome (SDS), sporadic olivopontocerebellar atrophy (sOPCA), and sporadic striatonigral degeneration. MSA was then subdivided into MSA-P (parkinsonism-predominant) and MSA-C (cerebellar-predominant).

### Epidemiology
- Prevalence is about 4 per 100 000.
- Typical age at onset is 55–60. Onset prior to age 30 has never been reported. Virtually all cases are sporadic; familial MSA is extremely rare.
- Males and females are equally affected.
- In most populations, about two-thirds of patients have MSA-P and one-third MSA-C, but these ratios are reversed in the Japanese.
- Survival times for both types are similar: mean of 6–9 years from symptom onset. Functional disability generally occurs earlier in MSA-P.

### Pathology
The pathological hallmark of MSA is glial cytoplasmic inclusions containing alpha-synuclein, mainly found in the basal ganglia, cerebellar structures, and motor cortex.

### Clinical features
- In MSA-P, characteristic features are parkinsonism (usually poorly responsive to levodopa) with signs of autonomic failure: postural drop in blood pressure of >30 mmHg systolic/15 mmHg diastolic, urinary incontinence or incomplete bladder emptying, and erectile dysfunction (see Video 4.2: MSA).
- In MSA-C, cerebellar signs (jerky pursuit, nystagmus, dysarthria, dysmetria, gait ataxia) occur with autonomic failure.
- During disease progression, cerebellar signs often develop in patients with MSA-P, and parkinsonism in MSA-C.
- A number of other clinical features occur in MSA that are helpful in distinguishing it from other parkinsonian conditions. These may be present some years prior to the onset of parkinsonism or cerebellar signs. These 'red flags' include the following (for additional features, see p. 20):
  - early falls and postural instability (also seen in PSP)
  - dystonia affecting the orofacial muscles, occurring spontaneously or when levodopa treatment is initiated (also seen in PSP)
  - dystonia affecting the trunk and neck, leading to anterocollis and flexion of the trunk (Pisa syndrome—also seen in PSP)
  - jerky distal limb tremor due to stimulus-sensitive myoclonus
  - unusual quivering, high-pitched monotonous, or slurring dysarthria

- abnormal respiratory pattern with inspiratory sighs, stridor, sleep apnoea, and snoring
- RBD (→ p. 298). Also seen, but less common, in PD, and quite rarely in PSP
- cold hands and feet, Raynaud's phenomenon
- emotional incontinence: inappropriate crying/laughing (also seen in PSP)
- pyramidal signs (increase in reflexes, extensor plantar responses, but no weakness or scissoring of gait).

- Clinical features that would tend to exclude the diagnosis of MSA include dementia, hallucinations, positive family history, gaze paresis, clinically significant neuropathy, age of onset >75 years, extensive white matter changes on brain imaging.

### Clinical criteria for multiple system atrophy diagnosis

Clinical criteria for MSA diagnosis require[2] a progressive disorder with onset >30 years and:
- possible MSA: parkinsonism or a cerebellar syndrome AND at least one sign of autonomic dysfunction AND at least one of the additional features
- probable MSA: autonomic failure (urinary incontinence and erectile dysfunction OR orthostatic hypotension, e.g. 30 mmHg systolic, or 15 mmHg diastolic, drop after 3 minutes of standing) AND parkinsonism or a cerebellar syndrome
- definite MSA: pathology required.

#### Additional features
- For possible MSA-P or MSA-C:
  - Babinski sign with hyperreflexia, stridor.
- For possible MSA-P:
  - rapidly progressive parkinsonism; poor response to levodopa; postural instability within 3 years of motor onset; gait ataxia; cerebellar dysarthria; limb ataxia or cerebellar oculomotor dysfunction; dysphagia within 5 years of motor onset; atrophy on MRI of putamen, middle cerebellar peduncle, pons, or cerebellum; hypometabolism on 18-fluorodeoxyglucose (FDG)-PET in putamen, brainstem, or cerebellum.
- For possible MSA-C:
  - Parkinsonism (bradykinesia and rigidity); atrophy on MRI of putamen, middle cerebellar peduncle, or pons; hypometabolism on FDG-PET in putamen; pre-synaptic nigrostriatal dopaminergic denervation on SPECT or PET.

---

2 Gilman S, Wenning GK, Low PA, et al. (2008). Second consensus statement on the diagnosis of multiple system atrophy. *Neurology*, 71(9), 670–6.

## Investigations

There are no diagnostic tests for MSA, but certain investigations can offer support for the diagnosis.
- **Cardiovascular autonomic function tests**: these may also be abnormal in PD, but severe abnormalities within the first 5 years of symptoms are frequent in MSA and infrequent in PD.
- **Sphincter electromyography (EMG)**: EMG of the external anal sphincter shows denervation due to degeneration of the Onuf's nucleus in MSA, but also in many cases of PSP, and even some with PD. However, a normal result would be very unusual in MSA. Today, this test is not commonly used in clinical practice.
- **Structural imaging** (Figs. 4.2, 4.3, 4.4): degeneration of the middle cerebellar peduncles and pons can cause a cruciform appearance in the pons on axial MRI slices: the 'hot cross bun sign'. There may be putaminal atrophy and hypointensity and a hyperintense lateral 'slit-like' rim to the putamen. There may be cerebellar atrophy and hyperintensity of the middle cerebellar peduncles. Putaminal, middle cerebellar peduncle, pons, or cerebellar atrophy on MRI are considered as additional features supporting the diagnosis of possible MSA in the currently used clinical criteria (➜ p. 103). DWI MRI may show high diffusion in the putamen in MSA and PSP, but not in PD.
- **Functional imaging**: DAT scans are abnormal in MSA, PSP, and PD. MIBG scintigraphy is abnormal in PD because of post-ganglionic sympathetic denervation but is typically normal in MSA (cardiac dysautonomia in MSA is due to central autonomic failure). IBZM is normal in PD, and abnormal in MSA (but also PSP and CBD). FDG-PET shows hypometabolism in the putamen, pons, and cerebellum, and is also considered as an additional feature in the criteria for possible MSA (see Clinical criteria for multiple system atrophy, ➜ p. 103).

## Treatment

- **Parkinsonism**: many patients with MSA show some levodopa response, but this may be short-lived, may cause cranio-cervical dystonia, and may worsen postural hypotension. Amantadine may be helpful for gait disturbance.
- **Orthostatic hypotension**: head-up tilt to bed at night, high-salt diet, elastic compression stockings; avoid hypotensive drugs, alcohol, or large meals.
- Pharmacological measures include ephedrine 15–45 mg tds, fludrocortisone 100–300 micrograms daily, midodrine (alpha-receptor agonist) 2.5–7.5 mg tds (all of these are available, but not licensed for this indication, in the UK).
- **Urinary dysfunction**: assessment with urodynamics is essential to characterize the nature of bladder dysfunction. Oxybutynin can be helpful for detrusor hyperreflexia, and intermittent self-catheterization is helpful for those with a large residual volume. Desmopressin can be helpful for nocturnal polyuria.

- **Erectile dysfunction**: sildenafil may be efficacious but can dramatically worsen postural hypotension. Intracavernosal injections of alprostadil (prostaglandin E1) or penile implants may be effective, without worsening hypotension.
- **Emotional incontinence**: may be helped by SSRIs or tricyclic antidepressants.

### Conditions confused with multiple system atrophy: the MSA lookalike syndromes

| Hereditary and sporadic neurodegenerative disorders | Parkinson's disease |
|---|---|
| | Progressive supranuclear palsy (in particular PSP-P), corticobasal degeneration, dementia with Lewy bodies |
| | Neurofilament inclusion body disease |
| | Spinocerebellar ataxias (SCA 1, 2, 3, 6, 7) |
| | Fragile X-associated tremor/ataxia syndrome (FXTAS, *FMR1* pre-mutation carriers) |
| | Prion (rarely) |
| | Vascular parkinsonism |
| | Primary progressive multiple sclerosis |

## Imaging in multiple system atrophy

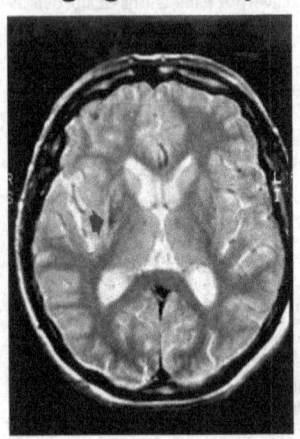

**Fig. 4.2** Putaminal atrophy, hyperintense rim (arrow), and putaminal hypointensity in comparison with the globus pallidus on T2-weighted images (1.5 T) in a patient with multiple system atrophy.

Reproduced from *J Neurol Neurosurg Psychiatry*, **65**(1), Schrag A et al., Clinical usefulness of magnetic resonance imaging in multiple system atrophy, pp. 65–71, Copyright (1998), with permission from BMJ Publishing Group Ltd.

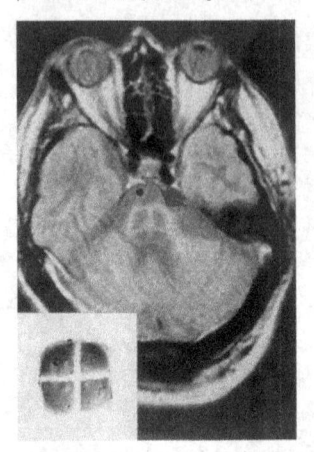

**Fig. 4.3** T2-weighted images (0.5 T) in a patient with pathologically proven multiple system atrophy showing infratentorial atrophy and signal change in the pons (cross sign, arrow), resembling a hot cross bun (inset).

Reproduced from *J Neurol Neurosurg Psychiatry*, **65**(1), Schrag A et al., Clinical usefulness of magnetic resonance imaging in multiple system atrophy, pp. 65–71, Copyright (1998), with permission from BMJ Publishing Group Ltd.

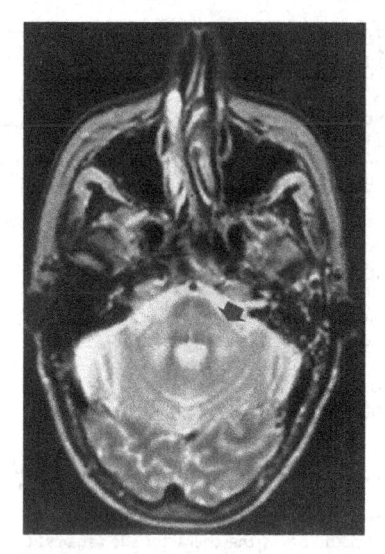

**Fig. 4.4** Infratentorial atrophy and signal change in the pons, middle cerebellar peduncles (arrow), and cerebellum on T2-weighted images (0.5 T) in a patient with multiple system atrophy.

Reproduced from *J Neurol Neurosurg Psychiatry*, 65(1), Schrag A et al., Clinical usefulness of magnetic resonance imaging in multiple system atrophy, pp. 65–71, Copyright (1998), with permission from BMJ Publishing Group Ltd.

# Corticobasal degeneration

CBD was first described in 1968 by Rebeiz and colleagues, as a syndrome of progressive slowness and stiffness in the limbs, dystonia, numbness or 'deadness' of the affected limbs, and gait disturbance. The condition has gone by a number of names in the past, including corticonigral degeneration with neuronal achromasia, cortical degeneration with swollen chromatolytic neurons, and corticobasal ganglionic degeneration (see Video 4.3: CBD).

## Epidemiology

- Prevalence is unknown, but considerably less than that of PSP or MSA.
- Males and females are equally affected.
- Average age at onset is 63, with youngest age at onset reported as 45.
- Average time from symptom onset to death is 8 years.
- CBD is almost always a sporadic condition, although a few familial cases with pathological confirmation have been reported.

## Pathology

CBD is characterized by widespread deposition of hyperphosphorylated tau protein (specifically 4-repeat tau) in the brain. There is marked neuronal degeneration in the substantia nigra and the fronto-parietal cortex. The hallmark feature of CBD pathology is the characteristic astrocytic plaques that differentiate CBD from other 4R tauopathies such as PSP (tufted astrocytes).

## Clinical features

### Motor symptoms

Patients typically present with asymmetrical rigidity and bradykinesia affecting one limb. Progressive dystonia often also affects the limb. The limb is often described by the patient as 'dead' or 'useless' and is frequently held postured across the body. Myoclonus (distal, stimulus-sensitive) often occurs. 'Alien-limb phenomena' occur where the affected limb seems to have a mind of its own, occurring in up to 50% of patients. Without the patient willing it (or sometimes even noticing it), the limb may move about, often grabbing objects or interfering with the actions of the 'good' hand (intermanual conflict).

### Cortical dysfunction

Apraxia is a cardinal clinical feature of CBD. It can be difficult to demonstrate in the more affected arm because of severe bradykinesia, rigidity, and dystonia. However, it is usually also present in the 'good' arm. Patients will often have cortical sensory loss (impaired 2-point discrimination, dysgraphaesthesia, astereognosis).

Dementia is an important part of the phenotype and may be the presenting or predominant clinical feature. Neuropsychometry typically reveals frontal executive defects, together with parietal lobe dysfunction. In contrast with Alzheimer's disease, episodic memory is usually well preserved.

## Eye signs

Patients with CBD may have difficulty in initiating saccades, but, once initiated, they are usually of normal velocity, which is the converse of most PSP subjects, but there is considerable overlap.

## Corticobasal degeneration phenotypes

The classical CBD phenotype (that is the combination of an asymmetric parkinsonian syndrome with cortical signs) is now called corticobasal syndrome (CBS). However, further phenotypes of patients with CBD pathology have been described. CBD may present with an FTD, PSP-RS, primary progressive aphasia, or a posterior cortical atrophy syndrome. Conversely, patients with other pathologies, such as Alzheimer's disease, PSP, and FTD pathology, may present with CBS.

## Clinical criteria for corticobasal degeneration

There are several sets of criteria for the diagnosis of CBD with low sensitivity and specificity. Recently, new clinical criteria have been proposed[3] that take into account the different phenotypes. None of the proposed sets of criteria have been prospectively validated.

## Investigations

There are no diagnostic tests for CBD. The following investigations may be of help in the differential diagnosis.
- **Structural imaging**: later in the course of CBD, asymmetric fronto-parietal atrophy may be seen.
- **Functional imaging**: DAT scans are typically abnormal in CBD, as they are in PD, PSP, and MSA. Glucose metabolism, measured by FDG-PET, and blood flow, measured by SPECT scanning, may show asymmetric reduction in fronto-parietal regions in CBD. This is not a feature typically seen in PSP, MSA, or PD.

## Treatment

- Treatment options for motor symptoms are very limited. A trial of levodopa is worthwhile, but rarely effective. Amantadine may be helpful for parkinsonism and gait disturbance. Valproate or levetiracetam may help myoclonus.
- BT injections can be helpful to relieve dystonic spasms of the hand—'the dystonic clenched fist'. These injections do not restore function but can help with hand hygiene and pain.
- No trials of cholinesterase inhibitors for dementia in CBD currently exist.
- Early management of dysphagia is important. Prompt provision of walking aids or a wheelchair can help prevent falls.

---

3 Armstrong MJ, Litvan I, Lang AE, et al. (2013). Criteria for the diagnosis of corticobasal degeneration. *Neurology*, **80**(5), 496–50.

**Conditions confused with corticobasal degeneration (presenting with corticobasal syndrome): the CBD lookalike syndromes**

- Progressive supranuclear palsy (accounts for the vast majority of misdiagnosis)
- Dementia with Lewy bodies
- Parkinson's disease
- Other dementias, e.g. Alzheimer's disease, Pick's disease, fronto-temporal dementia linked to chromosome 17q (FTDP-17), and genetic fronto-temporal dementias (*C9ORF72*, *PGRN*, *MAPT*, *FUS* mutations)
- Perry syndrome (*DCNT1* mutations)
- Cerebrovascular disease
- Progressive leukoencephalopathy with axonal spheroids (*CSF1R* mutations)
- Progressive multifocal leukoencephalopathy (very rare)
- Sudanophilic leukodystrophy (very rare)
- Prion disease (very rare)
- Neurofilament inclusion disease (very rare)
- Neurometabolic disorders (Gaucher's disease, cerebrotendinous xanthomatosis)

# Differentiating Parkinson's disease, multiple system atrophy, progressive supranuclear palsy, and corticobasal degeneration

|  | Parkinson's disease | Multiple system atrophy | Progressive supranuclear palsy | Corticobasal degeneration |
|---|---|---|---|---|
| Mean age at onset | 60 | 57 | 63 | 63 |
| Youngest reported onset | Childhood | 31 | 43 | 45 |
| Family history | Possible, particularly if onset <50 years | Virtually never | Very rare | Very rare |
| Symmetry | Asymmetric | Asymmetric | Symmetric | Asymmetric |
| Eye movements | Normal | May have square-wave jerks, jerky pursuit, nystagmus | Slowed vertical saccades, supranuclear gaze palsy | Delayed initiation of saccades |
| Dementia | Yes, usually late | Rare | Yes, frontal, prominent feature | Yes, prominent feature |
| Tremor | Often present | Often present, rarely pill-rolling | Uncommon | Jerky |
| Falls | May occur after some years of symptoms | Common early in course of disease | Very common early in course of disease | Common early in course of disease |
| Levodopa response | Good, prolonged, may develop dyskinesia | May cause dystonia, no prolonged response | Occasional response, not usually prolonged | Very occasional, short-lived response |
| Cardiovascular autonomic failure | May develop, but often late in disease | Often a prominent early feature | Very rare | Very rare |

*(Continued)*

|  | Parkinson's disease | Multiple system atrophy | Progressive supranuclear palsy | Corticobasal degeneration |
|---|---|---|---|---|
| Bladder disturbance | Urgency, frequency; incontinence secondary to immobility | Urgency, frequency, incontinence, incomplete bladder emptying | Urgency, frequency, incontinence, incomplete bladder emptying | Urgency, frequency; incontinence secondary to immobility |
| Other features | REM sleep behaviour disorder | Myoclonus, stridor, REM sleep behaviour disorder | Levator inhibition | Apraxia, cortical sensory loss, myoclonus, alien limb |

## Investigations

|  | Parkinson's disease | Multiple system atrophy | Progressive supranuclear palsy | Corticobasal degeneration |
|---|---|---|---|---|
| Olfactory testing | Usually abnormal | Usually normal | Usually normal | Usually normal |
| Levodopa challenge | Usually positive | May be positive | Rarely positive | Rarely positive |
| Cardiovascular autonomic function tests | Usually normal in early disease, may be abnormal later | Often abnormal early in the course of disease | Usually normal | Usually normal |
| Sphincter EMG | Usually normal | Rarely normal | Often abnormal | ? |
| Structural imaging | Normal | May have putaminal abnormalities, pontine 'hot cross bun', or cerebellar atrophy | May have midbrain atrophy or high signal, red nucleus atrophy, pallidal high signal | May have asymmetric fronto-parietal atrophy |
| DAT scan | Abnormal | Abnormal | Abnormal | Abnormal |
| Fluorodopa PET scan | Abnormal | Abnormal | Abnormal | Abnormal |
| Fluorodeoxyglucose PET | Usually normal | Impaired striatal uptake | Impaired striatal uptake | May show asymmetric fronto-parietal reduction in signal |

# Mechanisms of neurodegeneration

Abnormal folding and accumulation of protein is the common pathological mechanism underlying the development of a number of degenerative causes of parkinsonism, including PD, PSP, MSA, and CBD. The type of protein that accumulates (either tau or alpha-synuclein) and the main sites of accumulation are different in these conditions, which accounts for some of the clinical differences between them. Accumulation of misfolded protein is toxic to neurons and drives their degeneration.

## Tau and alpha-synuclein

Tau is a protein that is integral to the development and stability of microtubules, and therefore is important in axonal transport. There are six different forms (isoforms) divided into two main groups: 3-repeat tau (three copies of an amino acid sequence at the carboxy-terminal end of the protein) or 4-repeat tau (four copies of the same sequence). In the normal human brain, there is a balance between the amount of 3- and 4-repeat tau.

Alpha-synuclein is a protein of unknown function expressed pre-synaptically. The alpha-synuclein gene is mutated/overexpressed in two rare autosomal dominant forms of PD (*PARK1*, *PARK4*).

## Tauopathies and alpha-synucleinopathies

Degenerative causes of parkinsonism can be divided into those where misfolded alpha-synuclein is found or misfolded tau. Tauopathies can be further divided into those where there is an excess of 3-repeat or 4-repeat tau (Table 4.2).

Table 4.2 Tauopathies and alpha-synucleinopathies that cause degenerative parkinsonism

| Alpha-synucleinopathies | Tauopathies |
| --- | --- |
| Parkinson's disease | Progressive supranuclear palsy (4-repeat tau) |
| Dementia with Lewy bodies | Corticobasal degeneration (4-repeat tau) |
| Multiple system atrophy | Fronto-temporal dementia parkinsonism linked to chromosome 17 (3- and 4-repeat tau) |
|  | Globular glial tauopathies (4-repeat tau) |

## Mechanism of alpha-synuclein spreading

Recent evidence suggests the possibility that alpha-synuclein is a prion-like protein and that PD is a prion-like disease. Autopsy studies of patients with advanced PD who received transplantation of fetal nigral mesencephalic cells more than a decade earlier demonstrated that typical Lewy pathology had developed within grafted neurons, suggesting that alpha-synuclein had migrated from affected to unaffected neurons. Laboratory studies confirm that alpha-synuclein can transfer from affected to unaffected nerve cells where it appears that the misfolded protein can act as a template to promote misfolding of host alpha-synuclein. This leads to the formation of larger aggregates, neuronal dysfunction, and neurodegeneration. Indeed, recent reports demonstrate that a single intracerebral inoculation of misfolded alpha-synuclein can induce Lewy-like pathology in cells that can spread from affected to unaffected regions and can induce neurodegeneration with motor disturbances in both transgenic and normal mice. These findings support the hypothesis that alpha-synuclein may be a prion-like protein that can adopt a self-propagating conformation that causes neurodegeneration.

# Other degenerative causes of parkinsonism

Many degenerative disorders that cause parkinsonism are discussed elsewhere: Huntington's disease (HD; ➔ p. 164), X-linked dystonia parkinsonism (Lubag) (➔ p. 218), fragile X-associated tremor/ataxia syndrome (FXTAS; ➔ p. 286), neuroacanthocytosis (➔ p. 194), dentatorubropallidoluysian atrophy (DRPLA; ➔ p. 187), neuronal brain iron accumulation syndromes (NBIAs; ➔ p. 224), spinocerebellar ataxias (SCA; ➔ p. 282), and rapid-onset dystonia parkinsonism (RODP; ➔ p. 218).

## Basal ganglia calcification

Basal ganglia calcification confined to the globus pallidus is a common normal finding associated with ageing. However, calcification spreading outside this area may be associated with parkinsonism. Such calcification is best seen on CT. On MRI, it appears hypointense, similar in appearance to iron deposition.

### Causes of basal ganglia calcification that may cause parkinsonism

- Idiopathic basal ganglia calcification (IBGC or Fahr's syndrome): autosomal dominant basal ganglia calcification, presenting in the third or fourth decade with progressive parkinsonism, dystonia, tremor, dementia, and neuropsychiatric features such as psychosis. Two genes have been identified to cause autosomal dominant IBGC, namely, *SLC20A2* and *PDGFRB*. Rare autosomal recessive families have been reported, some with linkage to chromosome 14q.
- Secondary Fahr's syndrome:
  - hypoparathyroidism, pseudohypoparathyroidism, pseudo-pseudohypoparathyroidism
  - mitochondrial disease
  - post-infectious (usually congenital infection)
  - post-traumatic.

*Other causes of basal ganglia calcification*
- Cockayne's syndrome.
- Aicardi–Goutieres syndrome.
- Spinocerebellar ataxia 20 (dark dentate disease) (no gene identified).
- Haw River with DRPLA (➔ p. 187).

## Fronto-temporal dementia with parkinsonism

A number of autosomal dominant kindreds have been described, with a variable combination of parkinsonism, vertical gaze palsy, dystonia, and frontal dementia. In some, linkage has been demonstrated to chromosome 17 (*MAPT* gene, fronto-temporal dementia with parkinsonism linked to chromosome 17 (FTDP-17)). Pathologically, cases are characterized by tau-positive cytoplasmic inclusions, and many clinical similarities exist between FTDP-17, PSP, and CBD.

A recent breakthrough in the genetics of FTD was the identification of several genes causing FTD–amyotrophic lateral sclerosis overlap syndromes, namely the *C9ORF72* gene, and these patients may also have atypical parkinsonism; further identified genes causing FTD can also cause atypical parkinsonism such as *PGRN* gene mutations. Both *C9ORF72* and *PGRN* have TDP-43 pathology. Fused-in-sarcoma (*FUS*) mutations or pathology have also been linked to FTD atypical parkinsonism phenotypes.

## Perry syndrome

Perry syndrome is a rare autosomal dominant disorder due to mutations in the dynactin (*DCTN1*) gene, underpinned pathologically by TDP-43 inclusions. The age of onset ranges from 30 to 61 years. The penetrance is close to 50%. The typical phenotype includes parkinsonism, with varying combinations of central hypoventilation, weight loss, and psychiatric symptoms (e.g. apathy, hallucinations). Response to levodopa varies from no response to significant improvement and development of motor fluctuations and dyskinesias. However, Perry syndrome has been increasingly recognized to present with atypical features (PSP or CBS lookalikes).

## Pallidal degeneration syndromes

Some patients may present with striking progressive bilateral atrophy of the pallidum, sometimes combined with atrophy of other structures within the basal ganglia. Most cases are sporadic, although autosomal recessive inheritance is sometimes seen. Patients typically present with symmetrical parkinsonism, with a variable combination of dystonia, chorea, and myoclonus. Kufor–Rakeb syndrome (*PARK9*) is an autosomal recessive syndrome of pallidal and pyramidal atrophy, presenting in teenage years with vertical gaze palsy, parkinsonism, spasticity, and dementia. It is due to loss-of-function mutations in the *ATP13A2* gene, a mainly neuronally expressed ATPase of unknown function.

## Parkinson's disease–amyotrophic lateral sclerosis complex of Guam

Over 30 years ago, residents of the Pacific island of Guam were identified to have a particularly high incidence of PD, amyotrophic lateral sclerosis (ALS), and dementia, often occurring in the same patients. The incidence has gradually declined over time. It has been suggested that ingestion of the cycad plant during the Japanese occupation of the island in the Second World War (when other foodstuffs were scarce) resulted in long-term toxic effects on the nervous system.

### Neuronal intranuclear inclusion disease

Neuronal intranuclear inclusion disease (NIID) is a rare degenerative condition, characterized by the young onset (often in teenage years) of progressive parkinsonism, dystonia, ataxia, oculogyric crisis, autonomic failure, neuropathy, and dementia. Clinical features are highly variable. Levodopa response may be seen. The pathological hallmark is of eosinophilic inclusions within the nuclei of neurons. Diagnosis is possible in life with a full-thickness rectal biopsy where neurons will show characteristic inclusions. Recently, it has been shown that skin biopsy is also useful in diagnosing NIID, showing intranuclear inclusions stained positive with anti-ubiquitin and anti-SUMO1 antibodies in adipocytes, fibroblasts, and sweat gland cells.

### Neuronal intermediate filament inclusion disease

An uncommon neurodegenerative condition presenting as early-onset, sporadic FTD, associated with atypical parkinsonism and pyramidal signs, in instances resembling rapid-progression CBS. The neuropathology is characterized by neuronal inclusions that are immunoreactive for intermediate filaments (IFs), light, medium, and heavy neurofilament subunits, and alpha-internexin. Recently, abnormal intracellular accumulation of fused-in-sarcoma (FUS) protein has been found in a subgroup of neuronal intermediate filament inclusion disease (NIFID) patients.

# Secondary causes of parkinsonism

Many secondary disorders which cause parkinsonism are discussed elsewhere: WD (➔ p. 220), GM1 gangliosidosis (➔ p. 218), and drugs, including DRBs (➔ p. 253).

## Vascular parkinsonism

The first suggestion of a link between atherosclerosis and parkinsonism was made by Brissaud in 1895, and the term 'atherosclerotic parkinsonism' was coined by the neurologist MacDonald Critchley in 1929. There is persistent difficulty with the diagnosis of vascular parkinsonism: ischaemic damage to the basal ganglia is a very common finding in older individuals without parkinsonism, and therefore a causal relationship between ischaemic damage and parkinsonian symptoms is difficult to prove in individual patients. Typical features of vascular parkinsonism are as follows:

- sudden onset of symptoms and stepwise deterioration
- gait is severely affected early in the course of symptoms, with freezing and falls. In contrast, the upper limbs are relatively mildly affected. This pattern is called 'lower-body parkinsonism'
- upper motor neuron signs, including spasticity, brisk reflexes, extensor plantar responses, and pseudobulbar palsy
- cognitive impairment early in the course of disease
- poor response to levodopa
- vascular risk factors and history of vascular disease affecting other organs
- characteristic imaging findings are of deep subcortical infarcts. The basal ganglia may be peppered with small infarcts, described radiologically as a 'cribriform state'. DAT scans are typically normal but may be abnormal when on MRI the striatum is markedly involved
- pathological diagnosis relies on demonstration of vascular damage to the basal ganglia without the presence of Lewy bodies. In a neuropathological series, a much broader phenotype of vascular parkinsonism is revealed, which includes some patients with typical rest tremor, asymmetric signs, and response to levodopa.

## Toxins and parkinsonism

- Parkinsonism is associated with a number of toxins, including manganese, carbon monoxide, carbon disulfide, cyanide, methanol, organophosphates, and a variety of solvents.
- Manganese exposure occurs most often in welders, but also in battery makers, ore miners, and rarely in those with liver failure or those receiving total parenteral nutrition and in addicts injecting pseudoephedrine with potassium permanganate.
- Typical features of manganese toxicity include rapid development of symmetrical parkinsonism, dystonia, jerky tremor (often present during movement), behavioural disturbance, and cognitive impairment. A characteristic gait disturbance, known as the 'cock walk', occurs where the patient walks on tiptoes, with an extended trunk and arms held flexed at the sides.

- MR Imaging in manganism shows T1 hyperintensities within the basal ganglia, in particular the globus pallidus.
- A historically important toxic cause of parkinsonism is caused by MPTP, a compound that was produced as a toxic by-product of the synthesis of a heroin substitute by a 'designer drug' producer in California. A number of addicts who injected this compound in the late 1970s/early 1980s developed acute-onset parkinsonism. The parkinsonism is levodopa-responsive and is due to selective nigral neuronal damage, but Lewy bodies are not seen. MPTP is still of importance, as it is used to induce parkinsonism in animal models of PD.

## Infectious and post-infectious parkinsonism

### Encephalitis lethargica

This disorder was considered to be mainly of historical interest but more recently has re-emerged as a current, but rare, cause of parkinsonism. Coincident with influenza epidemics in the first half of the twentieth century, large numbers of patients developed a syndrome of ophthalmoplegia, oculogyric crises, sleep–wake inversion or somnolence, and behavioural disturbance. A number of these patients subsequently developed a parkinsonian syndrome—post-encephalitic parkinsonism. Such patients had a static, or very slowly progressive, syndrome of bradykinesia, rigidity, resting tremor, and gait disturbance, together with other features, including myoclonus, dystonia, supranuclear gaze palsy, and cognitive dysfunction. No clear link to the influenza virus has been established in encephalitis lethargica or post-encephalitic parkinsonism. Pathological studies found neurofibrillary tangles, but no Lewy bodies. Some limited levodopa response was noted in some patients.

More recently, a small number of patients with a post-infective encephalitis–lethargica-like clinical picture have been reported in the literature. Anti-basal ganglia antibodies (ABGAs) (➔ p. 146) have been reported in some of these patients, raising the possibility that prior streptococcal infection might be a precipitating cause in some patients.

### Other infections

Parkinsonism has been reported as a consequence of Japanese B encephalitis, Coxsackie B virus, measles, Epstein–Barr virus, and West Nile virus. Parkinsonism is also reported in human immunodeficiency virus (HIV) infection. Infective conditions which can cause focal lesions (e.g. cryptococcus, tuberculosis, and fungal infection) can cause parkinsonism via a direct lesion effect on the basal ganglia.

## Other

- Lesions of the basal ganglia due to infarct, tumour, demyelination, hypoxia, or infection can cause contralateral parkinsonism. The commonest site of such lesions is the substantia nigra.
- Parkinsonism can occur following repeated head trauma (older term: dementia pugilistica; current term: chronic traumatic encephalopathy), or secondary to hydrocephalus or severe head injury with midbrain compression.

# Useful websites and addresses

- **The PSP Association (UK)**: PSP House, 167 Watling Street West, Towcester, Northamptonshire, NN12 6BX. Tel: 01327 322410. www.pspassociation.org.uk Offers a nationwide network of PSP patient groups and a national helpline. The PSP Association also caters for patients with CBD. Cure PSP (USA); http://www.psp.org. Same aims as PSP Association above.
- **Multiple System Atrophy Trust (UK-formerly Sarah Matheson Trust)**: 51 St Olav's Court, City Business Centre, Lower Road, London, SE16 2XB. Tel:0333 323 4591; http://www.msatrust.org.uk. National organization catering for patients with MSA and other diseases causing autonomic failure. The MSA Coalition (USA - formerly the Shy Drager MSA Support Group); https://www.multiplesystematrophy.org/ Same aims as MSA Trust above.
- **International Parkinson and Movement Disorder Society**: http://www.movementdisorders.org. International movement disorders society.

# Chapter 5

# Tremor

Introduction *124*
Approach to the patient with tremor *126*
Rest tremor *128*
Postural tremor: 1 *130*
Postural tremor: 2 *132*
Other tremor syndromes *134*
Focal tremor syndromes *136*
Treatment of tremor *138*
Useful websites and addresses *140*

# Introduction

## Definition
Tremor is defined as a rhythmic sinusoidal oscillation of a body part. Usually this is due to alternate activation of agonist and antagonist muscles. This differentiates tremor from the jerks seen in myoclonus (→ p. 176) where this pattern of alternating muscle activity is not seen.

## Describing tremor

### Position
Clinically, the most useful way to categorize tremor is whether it occurs mainly at rest, on posture, or during movement (kinetic tremor). Some people prefer to call all tremors that do not occur at rest 'action tremors'. Action tremors are then subdivided into postural, kinetic (tremor during movement), and intention (tremor increasing throughout the movement). Terminal tremor—tremor occurring at the end of movement—is not synonymous with intention tremor and is seen in many kinetic tremors. We find the division into rest, postural, and kinetic tremor simpler and clinically more useful.

### Body part affected
Most tremors will affect the arms, and this will be the symptom that the patient complains of. However, some tremors are localized solely to other body parts such as the jaw, head, chin, or legs. Other tremor syndromes may present with a combination of limb tremor and tremor of other body parts, e.g. arm and head tremor in dystonia.

### Frequency
Tremor frequency is measured in hertz (Hz); a 3 Hz tremor has three cycles per second. EMG is a simple and quick method with which to calculate tremor frequency accurately.

### Amplitude
Unless specialist electrophysiological techniques are used, assessing the amplitude of a tremor is an essentially subjective process. However, it is clinically useful, and it is possible with experience, to divide tremors into those that are small-amplitude—usually called 'fine tremors'—and those that are large-amplitude. Some tremors, such as dystonic tremors, may have variable amplitude.

## Causes of tremor
Causes of tremor are listed in Table 5.1. They are divided into tremors that occur mainly at rest, in posture, or during movement, and body part-specific tremors such as head, chin, and jaw tremor. Some syndromes may cause combinations of rest, postural, and kinetic tremor. In such cases, the main tremor is listed, and other tremors that may occur are indicated in footnotes.

**Table 5.1** Causes of tremor

| | |
|---|---|
| Rest tremor | Parkinson's disease |
| | Drug-induced parkinsonism |
| | Vascular parkinsonism (rest tremor very rare) |
| | Progressive supranuclear palsy (rest tremor rare) |
| | Multiple system atrophy (<10% of cases) |
| | Spinocerebellar ataxia (esp. SCA 2, 3) |
| | Functional (psychogenic) tremor |
| Postural tremor | Enhanced physiological tremor |
| | Drugs* |
| | Toxins (mercury, toluene, solvents)* |
| | Metabolic disturbance (hyperthyroidism, Cushing's syndrome) |
| | Essential tremor |
| | Neuropathy* |
| | Dystonia* |
| | Task-specific tremors |
| | Parkinson's disease |
| | Multiple system atrophy (60% of cases) |
| | Spinocerebellar ataxia (esp. SCA 12) |
| | Fragile X-associated tremor/ataxia syndrome (FXTAS) |
| | Orthostatic tremor |
| | Functional (psychogenic) tremor |
| Kinetic tremor | Cerebellar disease (demyelination, haemorrhage, degenerative, toxic)† |
| | Holmes tremor† |
| | Wilson's disease† |
| | Functional (psychogenic) tremor |
| Head tremor | Essential tremor (uncommon) |
| | Dystonia |
| | Cerebellar disease (titubation) |
| | Third ventricular cysts (bobble-head doll syndrome) |
| | Spasmus nutans |
| | With congenital nystagmus |
| | Labyrinthine fistula |
| | As part of tic disorder |
| | Head banging in children |
| Chin tremor | Hereditary geniospasm |
| | Parkinson's disease |
| Jaw tremor | Parkinson's disease |
| | Dystonia |
| | Essential tremor (rare) |
| Palatal tremor | Essential |
| | Symptomatic |
| | With ataxia |
| | Functional (psychogenic) tremor |

* Rest component to tremor may also occur.
† Rest and postural components to tremor may also occur.

# Approach to the patient with tremor

## History
- Age at onset.
- Body part(s) affected.
- Sequence of body part involvement (e.g. hands, then neck, or neck followed by hands).
- Any precipitating factors at onset?
- Drug exposure (prescribed, illicit, alcohol, coffee, nicotine).
- Static or progressive course?
- Exacerbating factors (including if tremor is only present during a particular action, e.g. writing).
- Relieving factors (including response to alcohol).
- Associated neurological symptoms (e.g. slowness of movement, incoordination, sensory disturbance, limb weakness).
- Associated systemic symptoms (e.g. symptoms of hyperthyroidism).
- Family history of tremor (including site of tremor) or other neurological condition (including male mental retardation and premature ovarian failure).

## Examination
- Examine the patient at rest. Arms should be relaxed and ideally resting on the arms of a chair. If this is not possible, rest the patient's arms in their lap, half-pronated and relaxed. Ask the patient to perform a cognitive task (close the eyes and count backwards from 100) to bring out any tremor present.
- Examine the arms on posture. Ask the patient to stretch out their arms in front of them, with fingers spread a little, and to perform a cognitive task (close the eyes and count backwards from 100). Ask the patient to slowly flex the arms at the elbows and then slowly pronate and supinate the forearms, looking for exacerbation of tremor in particular positions.
- Examine the arms during movement. Ask the patient to touch their nose with their index finger and then the tip of the examiner's finger held at the extreme of their reach. Look for tremor that occurs during movement, tremor that worsens throughout movement (intention tremor), or tremor that only occurs as the target is approached (terminal tremor). Sometimes it is easier to detect dysmetria by doing a knee–ear lobe test, withdrawing visual feedback at the end of the trajectory.
- Ask the patient to write with their dominant hand and copy a spiral with both hands. This is useful to look for task specificity of tremor and also as a way of monitoring response to treatment.
- Is the movement disorder seen really a tremor, or might it be a myoclonus?

- Examine for other neurological signs, in particular parkinsonism, cerebellar signs, and signs of peripheral neuropathy.
- Examine for signs of systemic disease (e.g. signs of hyperthyroidism).

### Investigation
- Investigation is guided by the tremor type seen and any associated symptoms and signs. Often extensive investigation is not needed. Thyroid function tests may be indicated, and, in patients under 45 years, consider copper and ceruloplasmin (although normal results do not completely exclude WD; ➔ p. 220).

# Rest tremor

## Parkinson's disease
(See ➔ p. 26.)
- This is the commonest cause of a rest tremor.
- Typically, an asymmetric 3–4 Hz moderate-amplitude tremor involving the hand.
- The term 'pill-rolling' is often used to describe the tremor of PD. This is because the tremor often involves the thumb, and the patient appears to be rolling something between their thumb and index finger.
- Flexion tremor of the thumb is a very useful sign, as it is only rarely caused by conditions other than PD. However, extension thumb tremor may be seen in dystonic tremor.
- Other rest tremors occur in PD, including pronation/supination of the forearm, adduction/abduction of the leg, and jaw tremor. Head tremor is only very rarely seen.
- Rest tremor is usually worsened by a cognitive task, and tremor of the hand is often brought out by walking.
- Some patients with PD do not have tremor, while some patients with PD have tremor as their main symptom—'tremor-dominant PD'. There is a subgroup of patients with an older age of onset of symptoms (>70 years) who have tremor as their main symptom and a very slowly progressive course. These patients are sometimes categorized as having 'benign tremulous Parkinson's disease'.
- Other tremors may occur in PD (Box 5.1).
- Conditions that cause postural tremor, such as hyperthyroidism and drugs, can worsen tremor in PD (see Video 5.1: PD tremor).

## Other parkinsonian conditions
- Rarely, PSP (➔ p. 96) and MSA (➔ p. 102) can cause a rest tremor.
- DRBs (➔ p. 252), WD (➔ p. 220), and some SCAs, such as SCA 2 and 3 (➔ p. 282), can all cause parkinsonian signs, including a rest tremor.

## Other conditions
- Some tremor syndromes have a rest component, but a more prominent postural or kinetic tremor. These include dystonic tremor (➔ p. 132), neuropathic tremor (➔ p. 130), rubral tremor (➔ p. 134), and cerebellar tremor (➔ p. 134). Rhythmic myoclonus may mimic rest tremor.

## Investigation
- Rest tremor is most commonly caused by PD, and, in a typical clinical scenario, investigation is often not needed.
- In cases where the diagnosis is not clear, a DAT scan can be helpful. This is abnormal in PD and also in other conditions causing pre-synaptic loss of dopaminergic neurons (e.g. MSA and PSP).

However, DAT scans are normal in drug-induced parkinsonism, ET, and dystonic tremor.
- Blood testing for WD (→ p. 220) and structural brain imaging may be helpful.

#### Box 5.1 Tremors that may occur in Parkinson's disease
- **Rest tremor**: asymmetric, 3–4 Hz, moderate amplitude. Typically involves the thumb and index finger—'pill-rolling'. May involve other body parts, including the legs, jaw, and chin.
- **Postural tremor**: asymmetric, 6–8 Hz, moderate amplitude. Occurs immediately on stretching out the arms.
- **Re-emergent tremor**: asymmetric, 3–4 Hz, moderate amplitude. Occurs in patients with rest tremor. When they stretch their arms out in front of them, there is no tremor, but, after a few seconds, a rest tremor recurs (re-emerges) in the new position.

### Scans without evidence of dopaminergic deficit (SWEDDs)
- This term was originally coined when functional imaging of patients enrolled in drug studies for PD revealed that approximately 10% of patients had normal dopaminergic functional imaging.
- These patients (usually) presented with an asymmetric rest tremor that resembles PD tremor.
- In only a small number of cases, follow-up dopaminergic functional imaging became abnormal, whereas, in the majority, scans remained normal, even on long-term follow-up.
- The term was initially useful to highlight the existence of these patients but does not describe a specific entity, as these patients have diverse aetiologies for their symptoms.
- A specific group of these patients has been highlighted in the literature who have adult-onset asymmetric rest and postural tremor.
- Some of these patients have additional features of dystonia, and electrophysiological evaluation suggests features previously reported in patients with dystonia.

## Postural tremor: 1

ET and dystonic tremor are important causes of postural tremor that are considered separately on ➲ p. 132.

### Physiological tremor

A fine postural tremor is a normal phenomenon, and the intensity is subject to normal variation. Physiological tremor is enhanced by anxiety and fatigue. However, it is important not to dismiss a tremor as 'enhanced physiological tremor' without considering alternative diagnoses.

### Drugs and toxins

Drugs (prescribed drugs, illicit drugs, coffee, alcohol, nicotine) are very common causes of postural tremor (➲ p. 260). Therefore, a detailed drug history is essential, in particular to determine when a particular drug was started in relation to the onset of the tremor. Remember that many patients do not regard herbal remedies as drugs, and specific enquiry needs to be made about 'over-the-counter' drugs.

Toxins that can cause tremor include solvents and mercury. Hat makers used to use mercury and often developed tremor ('hatter's shakes') and psychosis (like the Mad Hatter in *Alice in Wonderland*).

### Metabolic disturbance

Hyperthyroidism is the most important metabolic cause of tremor, and thyroid function tests should be performed in all patients with otherwise unexplained tremor. Other metabolic causes of tremor include Cushing's syndrome and liver disease.

### Neuropathic tremor

- Peripheral neuropathy can cause postural tremor (and, to a lesser extent, rest and kinetic tremor).
- Tremor is particularly seen with the demyelinating sensorimotor neuropathy associated with immunoglobulin M (IgM) paraproteinaemia and anti-myelin-associated glycoprotein (anti-MAG) antibodies. However, tremor is often seen in other neuropathies, including hereditary sensorimotor neuropathy (HSMN) and chronic inflammatory demyelinating polyradiculoneuropathy (CIDP).
- Signs of peripheral neuropathy are almost always clearly present at the onset of the tremor, and treatment of the underlying neuropathy may improve the tremor.
- Neuropathic tremor is different from the abnormal movements that occur in pseudo-athetosis. Pseudo-athetosis occurs in limbs that have impaired proprioception. Abnormal movements (typically slow distal writhing movements) occur when the patient has their eyes closed but are abolished or improve on looking at the affected limbs.

### Other tremors

Fragile X syndrome (➔ p. 286), SCA such as SCA 12 (➔ p. 282), PD (➔ p. 26), WD (➔ p. 220), and familial cortical tremor (➔ p. 182) should be considered in the differential diagnosis of postural tremor.

### Tests to consider in the investigation of postural tremor
- Thyroid function tests
- Liver biochemistry
- Screening for Wilson's disease (➔ p. 220)
- Blood for measurement of heavy metals (e.g. mercury)
- Nerve conduction studies, serum protein electrophoresis, anti-MAG antibodies in patients with signs of peripheral neuropathy
- EMG to assess tremor frequency and to look for signs of myoclonus (familial cortical tremor; ➔ p. 182)
- Genetic testing for FXTAS, SCA (in particular SCA 12)

## Postural tremor: 2

### Essential tremor
- A syndrome of symmetrical postural or kinetic tremor that is often inherited in an autosomal dominant fashion.
- Onset is said to be bimodal. Childhood and senile onsets are well described. Men and women are equally affected. Prevalence is estimated to be approximately 300 per 100 000.
- Typical clinical presentation is with a fine distal symmetrical tremor of the arms at 8–10 Hz. It is rarely present at rest but may persist during movement. ET is usually of gradual onset and tends to worsen slowly over time. Minor head and voice tremor may occur.
- A beneficial effect of alcohol on the tremor is often seen.
- A dominant family history is often found—relatives may have been misdiagnosed as having PD.
- ET is thought to be due to the action of an abnormal central oscillator, probably located in the brainstem.
- Despite the strong autosomal dominant inheritance, no genes for the common variant ET have been discovered to date. Genetic linkage studies and a meta-analysis have confirmed an association with rs9652490 polymorphism in the *LINGO1* gene (leucine-rich repeat and Ig domain-containing 1).
- There are no diagnostic tests for ET. Exclusion of other causes of postural tremor (e.g. drugs, hyperthyroidism) and careful examination for signs of other movement disorders, such as dystonia or neuropathy, are important. Proposed diagnostic criteria are given in Box 5.2 (see Video 5.2: Essential tremor).

### Dystonic tremor
- Tremor is well recognized to occur as part of dystonia (→ p. 196). In many cases, the diagnosis is clear, as signs of dystonia (abnormal posture) will be present with the tremor. Often tremor will occur in the body part affected by dystonia (e.g. head tremor with dystonia affecting the neck), but it may occur in a body part unaffected by dystonia (e.g. arm tremor in patients with neck dystonia). Rarely, dystonic tremor may mimic PD tremor, which is the case, for example, patients with DAT scans labelled as SWEDDs.
- However, in some patients, signs of dystonia are minimal. In such cases, the main differential diagnosis is between dystonic and ET.
- Factors that can be helpful in determining between essential and dystonic tremor are given in Table 5.2. Dystonic tremor is often position-specific. Examination of the patient slowly pronating and supinating the arms can be helpful to look for this. Dystonic tremors are often made worse by particular tasks (e.g. writing).
- Task-specific tremors are probably a form of dystonic tremor. In these syndromes, tremor only or predominantly occurs during performance of a particular task.
- The commonest of these tremor syndromes is primary writing tremor where the patient experiences a tremor of the arm only when writing (see Video 5.3: Dystonic tremor).

**Table 5.2** Factors that help to distinguish between essential and dystonic tremor

|  | Essential tremor | Dystonic tremor |
| --- | --- | --- |
| Amplitude | Small and constant | Large and variable—sometimes described as 'jerky' |
| Symmetry | Symmetrical | Asymmetrical |
| Dystonia | Not present | Often present |
| Position specificity | Not present | Tremor often worse in particular positions |
| Task specificity | Not present | Tremor often worse in performance of particular tasks |
| Family history | Majority of cases | Not uncommon |
| Improvement with alcohol | Often dramatic | Can occur |
| Response to propanolol | Often good | Usually little response |

### Box 5.2 Movement Disorder Society criteria for diagnosis of essential tremor

#### Inclusion criteria
- Bilateral, largely symmetric postural or kinetic tremor involving the hands and forearms that is visible and persistent
- Possible additional or isolated tremor in the head, but absence of abnormal posturing

#### Exclusion criteria
- Other abnormal neurological signs, especially dystonia
- The presence of known causes of enhanced physiologic tremor, including current or recent exposure to drugs that are known to cause tremor or a drug withdrawal state
- Historical or clinical evidence of psychogenic tremor
- Convincing evidence of sudden onset or evidence of stepwise deterioration
- Primary orthostatic tremor
- Isolated voice tremor
- Isolated position- or task-specific tremors, including occupational tremors and primary writing tremor
- Isolated tongue, chin, or leg tremor

# Other tremor syndromes

## Kinetic tremor

### Cerebellar tremor
- The commonest cause of kinetic tremor is disease of the cerebellum or its outflow pathways.
- The typical tremor in cerebellar disease progressively augments over the course of the movement.
- This tremor is called 'intention' tremor. It is revealed by performing finger–nose (or knee–ear) testing.
- Head tremor (titubation) is often present with cerebellar disease, as are other cerebellar signs, including saccadic pursuit, nystagmus, dysmetria (past-pointing), dysdiadochokinesia (irregular rate, force, and rhythm of alternating movements), rebound, heel–shin ataxia, and gait ataxia. Tremor and other cerebellar signs are all ipsilateral to the cerebellar hemisphere that is damaged.
- Common causes of cerebellar tremor include demyelination, ischaemic/haemorrhagic damage to the cerebellum, toxic effects of drugs and alcohol, heredo-degenerative diseases affecting the cerebellum or its connections (e.g. SCA syndromes), and paraneoplastic cerebellar degeneration (see Video 5.4: Cerebellar tremor).

### Holmes tremor
- This tremor syndrome is characterized by tremor that is present at rest, worse on posture, and much worse during movement. Named after the neurologist Gordon Holmes (1876–1965). Synonyms include rubral tremor and midbrain tremor.
- It is due to damage to cerebellar connections within the brainstem.
- A tremor of this type is characteristic of WD where a very violent 'wing-beating' tremor occurs during movement (see Video 5.5: Holmes tremor).

## Functional (psychogenic) tremor

Tremor is a common occurrence in functional movement disorders and is discussed in detail in Chapter 15 (➔ p. 318). Functional tremor may occur at rest, on posture, or during movement, or a combination of these (see Video 15.1: Psychogenic tremor).

## Tremor-mimic syndromes

A number of conditions can mimic tremor, most commonly disorders causing rhythmic myoclonus:

- Myoclonus (see ➔ Chapter 8):
  - positive rhythmic myoclonus (as in familial cortical tremor; ➔ p. 182)
  - negative myoclonus (as in asterixis)
  - spinal segmental myoclonus (➔ p. 190)
  - myoclonus secondary to root/plexus damage (➔ p. 190)
- Epilepsia partialis continua
- Stereotypies
- Other dyskinetic syndromes (e.g. hemifacial spasm, hemi-masticatory spasm; ➔ p. 310)
- Myorhythmia.

# Focal tremor syndromes

## Orthostatic tremor
- A tremor syndrome characterized by a fine, very high-frequency tremor of both legs. Tremor frequency is usually 16–18 Hz, although tremor at half this frequency (8–9 Hz) is also seen at other times.
- Patients usually complain of unsteadiness on standing, which is relieved by walking or sitting. In extreme cases, patients are unable to stand still and, if they cannot sit down, will be forced to pace around.
- As the tremor is of such high frequency, it may not be easy to see. It is best appreciated by the examiner placing his hands on the patient's legs while the patient is standing—a fast quivering of the legs may be felt. If a stethoscope is placed on the thighs, a noise, rather like a helicopter, might be heard.
- Postural tremor of the arms may also occur.
- In many patients, orthostatic tremor (OT) is an isolated phenomenon that does not progress, with typical age at onset of 50 years (primary OT). Other patients, usually with an older age at onset, may have other neurological signs (e.g. parkinsonism, restless legs syndrome (RLS)) and are called 'OT-plus'.
- Transient OT can be induced in normal subjects by unexpectedly pushing them off balance. Therefore, OT may be caused by damage to a central oscillator that normally acts to maintain balance. A pre-synaptic dopaminergic deficit has been found in some patients with primary OT.
- Clonazepam is sometimes beneficial, and a response to levodopa occurs in some patients.
- Some single case reports suggest this tremor may respond to thalamic DBS, but this has not yet been studied in a systematic fashion (see Video 5.6: Orthostatic tremor).

## Head tremor
- Head tremor is also known as titubation and is often described as 'yes–yes' (up and down) or 'no–no' (side to side).
- Common causes of head tremor include cerebellar disease and dystonia. Head tremor is only rarely seen in PD.
- 'Head bobbing' is a feature of third ventricular lesions (usually a cyst).
- Spasmus nutans is a childhood condition characterized by infantile onset of slow rhythmical head nodding with nystagmus and is usually self-limiting and of unknown aetiology. Head tremor may also accompany congenital nystagmus, aortic regurgitation, labyrinthine fistula, or 'neck shuddering' in tic disorders.

## Jaw tremor
- Often seen in PD and may be unresponsive to dopaminergic medication. Also seen in oromandibular dystonia or an isolated manifestation of dystonia. BT injections into the masseter can be helpful in these cases (see Video 5.7: Jaw tremor).

## Chin tremor

- May occur as an isolated symptom with autosomal dominant inheritance. It affects the mentalis muscle and is also known as hereditary geniospasm, or hereditary quivering chin. The responsible gene has been linked to an area on chromosome 9q13. May respond to BT injections.
- Chin tremor may also occur in PD.

## Palatal tremor

In this condition, rhythmic contraction of the muscles of the soft palate occurs at about 2 Hz. The patient may only complain of an annoying rhythmic clicking sound (which may be audible to others), caused by the opening and closing of the Eustachian tube by activation of the tensor veli palitini. Palatal tremor can be divided into essential (or isolated) and symptomatic forms. Palatal tremor was previously considered to be a form of rhythmic myoclonus but is more accurately classified as a tremor. Treatment options include clonazepam, sodium valproate, or BT. Palatal tremor may also be functional and can be diagnosed as such by applying current clinical criteria for functional movement disorders (see Video 5.8: Palatal tremor).

### Essential (isolated) palatal tremor

Palatal muscles are usually the only ones involved; ear clicking is common, and no lesion or secondary cause can be seen. The syndrome is non-progressive. Spontaneous resolution can occur but is rare.

### Symptomatic palatal tremor

Symptomatic palatal tremor is caused usually by activation of the levator veli palatini, and therefore ear clicking is less common than in the essential form. Adjacent muscles may be involved, including facial and masticatory muscles, ocular muscles, and cervical and upper limb muscles.

Most commonly, symptomatic palatal myoclonus is caused by a lesion within the Guillain–Mollaret triangle. This is an anatomical area within the brainstem formed by the ipsilateral inferior olivary nucleus, the ipsilateral red nucleus, and the contralateral dentate nucleus. Palatal tremor often develops some months after the original lesion. MRI can show bilateral inferior olivary hypertrophy.

A characteristic pattern of synchronous ocular, facial, and bulbar muscle spasm, which often includes palatal tremor (oculo-masticatory myorhythmia, OMM)), is seen in Whipple's disease. A progressive syndrome of palatal tremor with ataxia has also been reported (progressive ataxia palatal tremor syndrome, PAPT) and is described in detail in Chapter 12 (➔ p. 288).

# Treatment of tremor

## Treatment strategies
Treatment for the majority of tremor syndromes is purely symptomatic and is similar, regardless of the underlying cause of the tremor. Prior to commencing any treatment, it is essential to ask the patient if they feel that their tremor is disabling enough for them to want to try a daily treatment that may have side effects. Tremors associated with parkinsonism, in particular PD, may respond to dopaminergic therapy.

### Limb tremors
Except in cases of parkinsonism, treatment of limb tremor usually involves working through a list of medications that may be beneficial, trying each one in turn to the maximum dose tolerated, before proceeding to the next. This can be an arduous process for the patient (and doctor), and therefore a clear explanation of the need for this 'trial-and-error' approach is required.

A reasonable approach would be to try, in order, propranolol, clonazepam, primidone, topiramate, and gabapentin. For dystonic tremor, trihexyphenidyl would be appropriate as a first-line treatment. BT has a very limited role in the treatment of limb tremor, although it may be helpful for task-specific tremors, e.g. primary writing tremor.

### Focal tremors
BT can give excellent results in the treatment of focal tremors such as head, jaw, chin, and voice tremor. OT may respond to levodopa and clonazepam.

### Surgical treatment of tremor
For those with severe tremor, neurosurgery may be appropriate. Such treatment clearly requires specialist advice and counselling and carries potentially serious side effects. In tremor secondary to PD, DBS of the STN may treat the tremor and other parkinsonian symptoms. In other tremor syndromes, DBS of the ventro-intermediate nucleus (VIM) of the thalamus is used.

### Trihexyphenidyl (benzhexol)*
- Available as generic tablets 2 mg and 5 mg (white, scored), or in syrup (5 mg/5 mL).
- Starting dose is 1 mg daily. Increase by 1 mg every 4–7 days to reach 1 mg tds. Then increase by 1 mg every 4–7 days to reach 2–4 mg tds.
- If side effects occur, dose titration should be stopped and then re-attempted after 1–2 weeks. Maximum dose may, in some, usually younger, patients be as high as 50–100 mg daily.
- Common side effects: dry mouth, dry eyes, nausea, confusion, constipation, urinary retention.
- Important contraindication: closed-angle glaucoma.

### Propranolol*

- Available as generic (10 mg, 40 mg, 80 mg, 160 mg), (80 mg, slow release), (160 mg, slow release).
- Starting dose is 10–20 mg tds, or slow release 80 mg once daily.
- Dose should be increased by 30 mg every 2 weeks to reach 30–60 mg tds, if tolerated, or slow release 80 mg bd.
- Maximum dose 320 mg daily.
- Main side effects include postural hypotension, bradycardia, nightmares, insomnia, and impaired erections. Propranolol is contraindicated in those with a history of asthma or heart failure.

### Clonazepam

- Available in 500 micrograms (beige) or 2 mg (white) tablets. Tablets scored twice.
- Starting dose is 250 micrograms once daily (125 micrograms in the elderly).
- Increase every week by 250 micrograms to reach 500 micrograms to 1 mg bd or tds
- Maximum dose 4–6 mg daily.
- Main side effects are sedation, depression, and fatigue.

### Primidone*

- Available in 250 mg tablets (scored).
- Starting dose is 62.5 mg once daily. Increase by 62.5 mg every week to reach 250 mg bd or tds, if tolerated.
- Maximum dose 1.5 g daily
- Main side effects are sedation, ataxia, nausea, and rash. Elderly patients are very sensitive to side effects. Reduce the dose very slowly when withdrawing after chronic administration.

### Topiramate

- Available in 25 mg (light yellow), 100 mg (yellow), and 200 mg (salmon) tablets. Also as Topamax® Sprinkles (15 mg capsules).
- Starting dose is 25 mg daily. Increase by 25 mg every 1–2 weeks to reach 50–100 mg bd.
- Maximum dose 400 mg daily, although can go to 800 mg daily.
- Main side effects are sedation, poor memory, speech disturbance, nausea, abdominal pain, and weight loss. Acute myopia due to secondary closed-angle glaucoma has been reported, usually in the first month of treatment.

### Gabapentin

- Available as generic tablets of 100 mg and 400 mg, or as 100 mg (white) and 300 mg (yellow) capsules and 600 mg and 800 mg tablets.
- Starting dose is 100 mg once daily. Increase by 100 mg every 4 days to reach 300–600 mg tds.
- Maximum dose is 2.4 g daily (800 mg tds).
- Main side effects are sedation, dizziness, headache.

## Useful websites and addresses

- **National Tremor Foundation (UK):** Long Term Conditions Centre, Gubbins Lane, Harold Wood, Romford, Essex, RM3 OAR. Tel: 01708 386 399; http://www.tremor.org.uk.
- **International Essential Tremor Foundation (IETF):** PO Box 14005, Lenexa, KS 66285-4005, USA; http://www.essentialtremor.org.
- **International Parkinson and Movement Disorder Society:** http://www.movementdisorders.org.

# Chapter 6

# Tics

Introduction *142*
Approach to the patient with tics *144*
Primary tic disorders *148*
Gilles de la Tourette syndrome *150*
Treatment of Tourette's syndrome *152*
Secondary tic disorders *156*
Useful websites and addresses *158*

# CHAPTER 6 **Tics**

## Introduction

Tics are *involuntary, brief, stereotyped movements or vocalizations*. An important and clinically useful characteristic of tics is that they are *suppressible* by the patient for a short period of time. Typically, the patient will experience a growing feeling of anxiety and discomfort during tic suppression (premonitory urge) and, when allowed to relax, will release a flurry of tics. As tics are under a degree of voluntary control, it has been suggested that they should be called 'unvoluntary', rather than involuntary, movements. They typically involve the face, neck, and upper limbs.

Tics are very common—15% of the population will have a tic at some time. For the vast majority, this is a short self-limiting occurrence in childhood of little or no significance. However, in others, it heralds the start of a chronic tic disorder which may result in significant physical, psychological, and social disability.

### Classification of tics

- Tics can be **motor** (movement) or **vocal** (sounds).
- Motor tics can be *simple* (one discrete movement) or *complex* (combination of a number of movements) (Table 6.1).
- Vocal tics can be *simple* (single unarticulated sounds) or *complex* (stereotyped utterance of words or phrases) (Table 6.1).
- Other features that may be present are:
  - copropraxia—production of obscene gestures
  - echopraxia—copying the movements of others
  - coprolalia—saying obscene words
  - echolalia—copying the words of others
  - palilalia—repetition of the same phrase, word, or syllable (e.g. 'My name is Mark … k … k … k … k').
- **Stereotypies** are longer, sometimes complex, repetitive movements (e.g. body rocking, hand wringing) that are often performed for long periods of time at the expense of all other movements. A new definition for stereotypies has been recently suggested: a non-goal-directed movement pattern that is repeated continuously for a period of time in the same form and on multiple occasions and which is typically distractible.
- **Mannerisms** are unusual ways of carrying out a purposeful movement and may result from the incorporation of a stereotypy into normal voluntary movement.
- Tics can be classified as *primary* (idiopathic) or *secondary* to a variety of degenerative, structural, metabolic, and pharmacological causes.
- Primary tic disorders almost always start in childhood.
- True adult onset of tics is rare and is almost always due to a secondary cause. It is very important to ask the patient and relatives about possible tics in childhood or associated behavioural disturbance such as obsessionality and attention-deficit/hyperactivity disorder (ADHD). Many cases of apparent adult onset of tics in fact have evidence of tics in childhood.
- Tics associated with adult-onset primary dystonia have also been described.

**Table 6.1** Examples of simple and complex motor and vocal tics

|  | Motor | Vocal |
|---|---|---|
| Simple | Eye blinking, eyebrow raising, winking, forehead raising, pouting, nose wrinkling, shoulder raising | Grunting, sniffing, coughing, humming, whistling |
| Complex | Head shaking, touching self, touching others, kicking, jumping, hopping, copropraxia, echopraxia | Saying words or parts of words, coprolalia, echolalia, palilalia |

## Approach to the patient with tics

There are three main questions to answer in the history and examination of the patient with tics.
- Does the patient have tics or another movement disorder? (Box 6.1 gives a list of other phenomena that may be confused with tics. Here the duration and suppressibility are the most important factors to consider for the differential diagnosis of the movement disorder.)
- Is the tic disorder primary or secondary?
- What type of primary or secondary tic disorder is it? (Table 6.2 gives a list of primary and secondary causes of tics, which are described in more detail on subsequent pages.)

### Box 6.1 Movement disorders and other manifestations that need to be differentiated from tics
- Myoclonic jerks (not suppressible)
- Stereotypies (for definition, see ➔ p. 142)
- Epilepsia partialis continua (not suppressible, abnormal electroencephalography)
- Blepharospasm (in particular increased blinking)
- Hemifacial spasm (not suppressible, characteristic distribution, usually adult-onset)
- Startle syndromes
- Oculogyric crisis (longer and sometimes loss of consiousness)
- Palatal tremor/myoclonus

### History
- What was the age of onset of the tics? Patients may not recall the onset of tics, and therefore a collateral history from a relative is often very helpful.
- What are the movements and/or vocalizations that the patient has noticed?
- Were there any precipitating factors at onset (e.g. drugs, brain injury, and infection)?
- Is there a family history of a similar disorder or of a neurological disorder in general?
- Is there an associated psychopathology (e.g. OCD, ADHD, anxiety, depression, self-harm)?
- Are there any additional neurological past or current symptoms (e.g. dementia, epilepsy, peripheral neuropathy)?
- What is the nature and extent of any disability associated with the symptoms?

## Examination

- Are the tics suppressible? To check, explain to the patient that you would like them to stop all movements and sounds for 15–30 seconds. Assess their ability to suppress their movements and/or vocalizations. Ask the patient to describe their feelings during tic suppression.
- Motor tics, vocal tics, or both?
- Simple tics, complex tics, or both?
- Coprolalia/praxia, echolalia/praxia?
- Other movement disorders present (e.g. chorea, parkinsonism)?
- Other neurological signs (e.g. exaggerated startle response, peripheral neuropathy, cognitive disturbance)?

## Investigation

- Guided by history and examination findings. Usually no investigations are needed.
- In the right clinical context (see subsequent pages), consider copper studies, blood film for acanthocytes, anti-streptolysin O (ASO) titre, ABGAs, uric acid, genetic testing for HD and Rett's syndrome (females only), and brain imaging.

Table 6.2 Causes of primary and secondary tic disorders

| | |
|---|---|
| Primary tic disorders | Simple transient tics of childhood |
| | Chronic tics of childhood (>1 year) |
| | Gilles de la Tourette's syndrome |
| | Adult-onset tourettism |
| | Tics associated with primary dystonia |
| Secondary tic disorders | |
| Secondary to neurodegenerative disease | Huntington's disease |
| | Wilson's disease |
| | Neuroacanthocytosis |
| | Neuronal brain iron accumulation syndrome |
| | Fronto-temporal dementias (also stereotypies) |
| Secondary to developmental syndromes | Rett's syndrome |
| | Lesch–Nyhan syndrome |
| | Down's syndrome and other chromosomal abnormalities (Klinefelter's, XYY karyotype, Beckwith–Wiedemann syndrome) |
| | Fragile X |
| | Autism and autistic spectrum disorders |
| | Non-specific mental retardation |
| Secondary to structural brain lesions | Post-encephalopathy (e.g. perinatal anoxia) |
| | Basal ganglia lesions (usually caudate) |

(Continued)

**Table 6.2** (*Contd.*)

| | |
|---|---|
| Secondary to infections and/or immune-mediated | Sydenham's chorea |
| | ? Paediatric autoimmune neuropsychiatric disorder associated with streptococcal infection (PANDAS) |
| | ? Tics associated with anti-basal ganglia antibodies or surface dopamine-2 receptor antibodies |
| | Creutzfeldt–Jakob disease |
| | Paraneoplastic syndromes |
| | Anti-NMDA encephalitis (also stereotypies) |
| | Antiphospholipid syndrome |
| | Systemic lupus erythematosus |
| Secondary to drugs and toxins | Carbon monoxide poisoning |
| | Cocaine, amphetamines |
| | Methylphenidate |
| | Anticonvulsants (carbamazepine, lamotrigine, phenytoin) |
| | Dopamine receptor blockers (tardive tics) |

# Primary tic disorders

Primary tic disorders are characterized by the presence of tics, with no other neurological or systemic symptoms or signs, and no evidence of neurodegeneration or secondary cause. Almost all primary tic disorders have onset in childhood.

### Idiopathic simple transient tics of childhood

This is a common self-limiting disorder of children, affecting up to 15% of school-age children, more commonly boys than girls. The sole clinical feature is the presence of a *single simple motor or vocal tic*. Motor and vocal tics do not occur together, and multiple tics are not seen.

Symptoms may last up to a year, but often much less. It has been suggested that recent streptococcal infection may be a precipitating factor. Minor behavioural disturbance may accompany the motor symptoms. Investigation in typical cases is not needed, and treatment is simply reassurance of parents and child.

### Idiopathic chronic motor or vocal tic disorder

This category is used for children with single simple motor or vocal tics that persist for longer than a year. Consideration should be given to the diagnosis of Gilles de la Tourette syndrome (Tourette's syndrome, TS), as well as secondary causes of tic disorder. Patients with chronic motor or vocal tic disorder are often those who do not quite fit the diagnostic criteria for TS, but there may clearly be some overlap clinically.

### Gilles de la Tourette syndrome

Gilles de la Tourette syndrome is the most important primary tic disorder, in terms of disability caused, and is covered in detail on ➔ p. 150.

### Adult-onset tourettism

The diagnostic criteria for TS (➔ p. 151) explicitly state that onset of tics should be before age 18. However, some patients present with the adult onset of a TS-like clinical picture. On careful history taking, many of these patients will be found to have had tics or ADHD in childhood and can therefore be classified as having a recurrence of typical childhood-onset TS.

Most of the remaining patients will have a secondary cause for their tics, and appropriate investigation is important for any patient presenting with adult-onset tics. This leaves a very small group of patients who appear to have the adult onset of otherwise clinically typical idiopathic TS, for whom management is as for childhood-onset TS. These adult-onset patients often have severe symptoms, which can be rather refractory to treatment. Primary tics have been also reported in association with adult-onset primary dystonia. In the rare culture-specific startle syndromes (such as Latah; ➔ p. 330), startle-induced tics, coprolalia/praxia, and echolalia/praxia are commonly reported.

# Gilles de la Tourette syndrome

Gilles de la Tourette was a French neurologist of the late nineteenth century, and a pupil of Charcot. He described three patients with a combination of chronic psychiatric disturbance and tics starting in childhood. For convenience, the syndrome that bears his name is usually known as Tourette's syndrome (TS). This is perhaps a welcome shortening of his full name: Georges Albert Eduardo Brutus Gilles de la Tourette. Tourette led a colourful life, including surviving being shot in the neck by a patient, only to die some years later of dementia due to syphilis.

## Epidemiology

TS affects 0.5–1% of the population under the age of 18, and 0.3–0.5% of the adult population, reflecting that symptoms lessen or resolve in many patients with age. Males are more often affected than females (4:1).

## Pathophysiology

As would be expected for a neurodevelopmental disorder which frequently improves with age, functional and structural MRI has also shown defects in maturation of the corticosubcortical and corticocortical circuits regulating motor output control. The most consistent structural change in volumetric MRI studies is decreased volume of the caudate nucleus. Caudate volumes during childhood seem inversely correlated to tic severity in adulthood, supporting the role of the striatum as a core developmental abnormality underlying TS. The outward expression of Gilles de la Tourette syndrome is the tics themselves, but the internal experience of patients is often that of a sensory urge and sensitivity to environmental triggers to movement.

So as well as the traditional view of tics as resulting from defective inhibition of competing motor patterns, they can also be thought of as resulting from an inappropriate activation/selection of motor patterns. Functional MRI studies show increased activity in several cortical and subcortical regions (somatosensory, posterior parietal cortical regions, putamen, amygdala/hippocampus complex), while the caudate and anterior cingulate cortex show decreased activity during spontaneous tics. ABGAs (➔ p. 156) are commoner in TS (10–20%) than in the general population (2–5%), but the significance of this finding is unknown.

## Pathology of Gilles de la Tourette syndrome

Limited post-mortem studies suggest a reduced number, and an abnormal distribution, of interneurons in the caudate and putamen in Gilles de la Tourette. One of these interneuronal subtypes parvalbumin-positive, fast-spiking, gamma-aminobutyric acid Y-mediated (GABAergic) interneurons might modulate the surround inhibition necessary for focused choice execution.

## Genetics of Gilles de la Tourette syndrome

First-degree relatives have a 10- to 100-fold increased risk of developing the disorder. An autosomal dominant inheritance is seen in some patients with TS. Although multiple genes and chromosomal regions have been linked to Gilles de la Tourette, to date, no gene or common variant of major effect has been identified.

## Clinical features

The cardinal clinical feature of TS is the presence of multiple motor and vocal tics, with onset before the age of 18 (see Video 6.1: Tourette's syndrome). The current *Diagnostic and Statistical Manual of Mental Disorders (DSM)* V-TR criteria for diagnosis of TS include having two or more motor tics (e.g. blinking or shrugging the shoulders) and at least one vocal tic (e.g. humming, clearing the throat, or yelling out a word or phrase), although they might not always happen at the same time, that are present for at least a year. The tics can occur many times a day (usually in bouts) nearly every day. The disturbance must not be due to the direct physiological effects of a substance (e.g. stimulants) or a general medical condition (e.g. HD or post-viral encephalitis). Other clinical features include the following: echopraxia/lalia and palilalia. Coprolalia and copropraxia are uncommon (10%), despite their public notoriety.

- Non-obscene, socially inappropriate behaviours (NOSIs) are common, e.g. inappropriate non-sexual personal comments, 'You're wearing a horrible tie today doctor ... '
- Psychiatric disturbance. This is common, and often a major source of disability for patients with TS. Common psychiatric problems include:
  - ADHD
  - OCD
  - self-harm—may be as a complex motor tic, e.g. poking the eye with fingers or a sharp object
  - depression.

## Investigation

Where there is nothing to suggest a secondary cause, extensive investigation is not usually needed. Some patients require:
- copper, ceruloplasmin, acanthocytes
- formal assessment of any psychiatric co-morbidity.

Consider:
- brain MRI, uric acid
- genetic testing (HD, Rett's syndrome).

# Treatment of Tourette's syndrome

Only symptomatic treatment is available for TS. It is essential to determine which symptom(s) is the main source of disability. In some patients, psychiatric co-morbidity is the most disabling feature of TS, and treatment of this alone may be sufficient.

## Treatment of tics
- Dopamine receptor antagonists:
  - typical neuroleptics (haloperidol, pimozide): pimozide has a better side effect profile than haloperidol
  - atypical neuroleptics (D2, 5-HT2A and 2C blockade: risperidone, tiapride, sulpiride; D2, 5-HT1A and 2A blockade: amisulpride; monoamine depletor: tetrabenazine).
- A2 receptor antagonists (clonidine, guanfacine).
- Benzodiazepines (e.g. clonazepam).
- BT (particularly for vocal tics).
- Anticonvulsants (levetiracetam, topiramate); there are conflicting data regarding their effectiveness.
- Agents increasing histamine are currently under investigation.

## Treatment of associated psychopathology
- Cognitive behavioural therapy, 'habit reversal therapy'.
- For associated ADHD: clonidine, methylphenidate.
- For associated OCD: SSRIs.
- For associated depression: SSRIs.

## Treatment strategies
- Cognitive therapies can be effective in the treatment of TS and associated psychopathology and should be proposed, but their availability varies widely.
- Botulinum toxin injections are very useful in isolated or simple motor tics, as well as phonic tics, and offer a targeted intervention without systemic side effects. Interestingly, premonitory urge and sensations have been reported to also improve after repeated injections into the affected muscle group.
- Clonidine is effective against both tics and ADHD, and therefore is a rational first-line therapy in patients with both problems.
- DRBs are the mainstay of therapy for tics themselves. These drugs can cause acute and chronic movement disorders, and some affect QT interval, and therefore should be introduced with caution.
- Aripiprazole is now used more frequently than other drugs in the treatment of Gilles de la Tourette profile (2.5–5 mg/day), even though large double-blind studies are not available. Akathisia seems to happen more often than with other neuroleptics.
- Tetrabenazine, a dopamine-depleting drug, does not cause tardive dystonia/dyskinesia but can cause parkinsonism and depression.
- Risperidone, pimozide, or other neuroleptics could be introduced when the other treatments have failed and should be used with caution.

- Methylphenidate and similar drugs can worsen tics, but this should not prevent their use for treatment of ADHD in TS.
- Psychosurgery (e.g. anterior cingulotomy, thalamotomy) has been used in severely affected treatment-refractory patients, but no controlled trials are available.
- When patients are refractory to behavioural, pharmacological, and BT treatments, an emerging possibility is high-frequency (130–150 Hz) DBS. Clinical trials have targeted the thalamus, GPi, nucleus accumbens, STN, and GPe, with improvement, but there is no current consensus on the best target.

## How to introduce medications commonly used for the treatment of Tourette's syndrome

### Clonidine
- An alpha-2 receptor-blocking drug.
- Available in 100 micrograms tablets (scored).
- Starting dose is 50 micrograms bd.
- Increase every few days by 50 micrograms.
- Typical maintenance dose is 50–100 micrograms four times daily.
- Maximum dose 1.2 mg daily.
- Main side effects: bradycardia, sedation, dry mouth, headache.
- Sudden withdrawal may precipitate a hypertensive crisis.

### Aripiprazole
- A D2, and 5-HT1A and 5-HT2A blocking drug.
- Available in 5, 10, 15, and 30 mg tablets or oral solution.
- Starting dose 2.5–5 mg/day.
- Increase every few weeks by 5 mg.
- Typical therapeutic dose between 5 and 20 mg.
- Main side effects: drowsiness, agitation, weight gain, and sleep disturbances.
- Akathisia may be commoner than with other antipsychotics.

### Tetrabenazine
- Available in 25 mg tablets (yellow-buff, scored).
- Starting dose is 12.5 mg once daily.
- Increase every week by 12.5 mg to reach 12.5 mg tds, and then increase in 12.5 mg increments to reach 25–50 mg tds as symptoms require.
- Maximum dose 200 mg daily, but usually less than this is needed.
- Main side effects: parkinsonism, akathisia, and depression.

### Sulpiride
- Available as generic in 200 mg tablets and 200 mg/5 mL oral solution.
- Starting dose is 200 mg daily.
- Increase every 2–4 weeks by 200 mg.
- Usual maintenance dose is 400 mg bd.

- Maximum dose 1.6–2 g daily.
- Main side effects: extrapyramidal effects (parkinsonism, acute dystonic reactions, tardive dyskinesia/dystonia, akathisia), sedation, anti-muscarinic effects. Neuroleptic malignant syndrome is a rare, but important, side effect.

*Pimozide*
- Available in 4 mg tablets (green, scored).
- Starting dose is 2 mg daily.
- Increase, as required, by 2 mg every 2–4 weeks to reach effective dose.
- Normal maintenance dose is 6–8 mg daily.
- Maximum dose 20 mg daily.
- Main side effects: as for sulpiride. Pimozide may prolong QT interval and cause arrhythmias, and the Committee on Safety of Medicines (CSM) advice is for electrocardiography (ECG) prior to treatment. Long QT is a contraindication to treatment. Pimozide should not be given with other antipsychotic drugs or drugs that prolong the QT interval (e.g. tricyclic antidepressants).

## Secondary tic disorders

Secondary tic disorders may be of childhood or adult onset. 'Red flags' that point to the likelihood of a secondary tic disorder are given on ➲ p. 156. Symptomatic treatment of secondary tic disorders is similar to that of TS, with dopamine-depleting drugs and DRBs forming the mainstay of treatment (➲ p. 152). Common causes of secondary tic disorders are listed in Table 6.2 (➲ p. 145).

### Secondary tics associated with neurodegeneration

Important neurodegenerative causes of tics include HD (➲ p. 164), WD (➲ p. 220), NBIA (➲ p. 224), and neuroacanthocytosis (➲ p. 170). NBIA and neuroacanthocytosis can be of childhood onset and may produce a temporary confusion with TS or other idiopathic childhood tic disorders, before additional symptoms emerge. Tics and stereotypies may also be seen in dementia, in particular in FTDs.

### Secondary tics associated with mental retardation

- Tics and stereotypies are often seen in association with syndromes that produce mental retardation, including Down's syndrome, fragile X, and autism, as well as following perinatal brain injury.
- Rett's syndrome almost exclusively affects females (affected males usually die *in utero* or soon after birth). It causes developmental arrest and regression, with onset between age 1 and 2 years, stereotypic hand movements (usually described as 'hand wringing'), microcephaly, and sometimes seizures. The causative gene is the *MECP2* gene on the X chromosome.
- Lesch–Nyhan syndrome is a rare X-linked recessive disorder characterized by mental retardation, seizures, and abnormal movements, often manifest as self-mutilating behaviours (lip/tongue/finger biting). The condition is caused by deficiency of the enzyme hypoxanthine-guanine phosphoribosyltransferase (HPRT) and is associated with high plasma uric acid. Onset is usually in childhood, but rare cases with teenage, or even adult, presentation are reported.

### Secondary tics associated with structural lesions

Tics are a recognized consequence of brain injury (e.g. from stroke, tumour, demyelination, or hypoxia). Tics are most commonly associated with lesions of the caudate nucleus.

### Secondary tics associated with drugs

See ➲ p. 262.

### Secondary tics associated with infection

- Sydenham's chorea (SC) (➲ p. 172) may present with tics alone, or tics in combination with chorea or other movement disorders.
- PANDAS (paediatric autoimmune neuropsychiatric disorder associated with streptococcal infection) is a syndrome which has significant overlap with SC. Proposed criteria for diagnosis are:
  - presence of OCD and/or tics
  - paediatric onset

- episodic course with abrupt onset and dramatic exacerbations
- association with group A streptococcal infection
- association with neurological abnormalities such as adventitious movements, motoric hyperactivity, or chorea.

There is still an ongoing debate about PANDAS and problems with applying these criteria in clinical studies. A small placebo-controlled trial of intravenous immunoglobulin (IVIG) and plasma exchange in the treatment of these patients appeared to show benefit, but the study has been criticized for a number of methodological flaws.

- ABGAs (antibodies in the serum of patients that bind to a solution containing homogenized human basal ganglia from post-mortem donors) have been reported in patients with SC and have been identified in patients with tics (some fulfilling criteria for TS, some not). Controversy exists as to the pathogenicity of these antibodies and whether immune modulatory therapy might have a role in the treatment of ABGA-positive patients. No controlled trials exist to date.
- A number of further antibodies have been described to be positive in PANDAS cases such as anti-dopamine receptor, anti-tubulin, anti-lysoganglioside-GM1, and anti-pyruvate kinase antibodies, of which the significance is uncertain.

### 'Red flags' suggesting a secondary tic disorder

*History*
- Abnormal birth/development
- Cognitive decline
- Adult onset of tics
- Other neurological symptoms (e.g. seizures)
- Precipitant at onset (e.g. drugs, infection)
- Progressive course

*Examination*
- Neurological signs other than tics, in particular other movement disorders, pyramidal signs, peripheral neuropathy

# Useful websites and addresses

- Tourettes Action UK Postal address: The Meads Business Centre, 19 Kingsmead, Farnborough, Hampshire, GU14 7SR. Tel no: 01252 362 362638; Helpdesk 0300 777 8427; http://www.tourettes-action.org.uk Patient and family support and information.
- **Tourette Association of America**: http://www.tsa-usa.org. The official American TS association website.
- **Rett UK**: http://www.rettuk.org.
- **International Parkinson and Movement Disorder Society**: http://www.movementdisorders.org.

# Chapter 7

# Chorea

Introduction *160*
Approach to the patient with chorea *162*
Huntington's disease *164*
Genetics and genetic counselling in Huntington's disease *166*
Management of Huntington's disease *168*
Chorea and acanthocytosis *170*
Other causes of chorea *172*
Useful websites *174*

# CHAPTER 7 **Chorea**

## Introduction

### Definition

Chorea is defined as brief, irregular, purposeless movements that flit and flow from one body part to another. In essence, people with chorea appear constantly restless or fidgety.

The word chorea is a corruption of the Greek word *horos*—dance. It may have been coined by Paracelsus who used it to describe devotees of St Vitus, who, on his Saint's day, would dance maniacally in order to ensure good luck for the following year. Thomas Sydenham (➲ p. 172) gives a wonderful description of chorea:

> ... the hand can by no means be kept in the same posture for one moment ... if a cup of drink be placed into his hand, he represents a thousand gestures, like jugglers ... his hand being drawn hither and thither by the convulsion, he turns it about often for some time, till at length happily reaching his lips, he flings it into his mouth and drinks it greedily...
> 
> (Thomas Sydenham, 1624–1689)

Chorea is often generalized, but it may be confined to one region (e.g. the face) or one side of the body (hemichorea). In some cases, it can be difficult to distinguish chorea from tics or myoclonus. However, tics are suppressible for a prolonged period, and myoclonic jerks are very brief and do not flow throughout the affected part of the body as does chorea.

### Athetosis

Choreoathetosis is sometimes used as an alternative term to chorea. Athetoid movements are slow, mainly distal, writhing movements that are more correctly associated with dystonia than chorea. We recommend that the term choreoathetosis should be avoided and that the examiner should differentiate between chorea and the slower writhing movements that can be part of dystonia. If both are present, we favour the term choreodystonic.

### Ballism

This is severe proximal chorea where the patient experiences wild flinging movements of the affected limbs (📹 see Video 7.1: Ballism). Involvement of one limb is called monoballism, and of one side of the body is called hemiballism or hemiballismus. The cause is usually a vascular injury in, or near, the contralateral STN.

### Causes of chorea

Chorea has a wide differential diagnosis (Table 7.1). One way of trying to reduce the differential diagnoses and create a rational plan of investigations is to consider the causes of chorea by typical age at onset and typical character of onset (acute versus gradual). Therefore, in Table 7.1, causes are marked as to their typical character of onset (acute or gradual). Table 7.2 divides causes of chorea by typical age at onset (<18 years, >18 years, or variable).

**Table 7.1** Causes of chorea

| | |
|---|---|
| Inherited/degenerative disorders | Huntington's disease (HD)[†] |
| | HD-like syndromes[†] |
| | Wilson's disease[†] |
| | Neuroacanthocytosis[†] |
| | McLeod's syndrome[†] |
| | Dentatorubropallidoluysian atrophy (DRPLA)[†] |
| | Lesch–Nyhan syndrome[†] |
| | Benign hereditary chorea[†] |
| | Ataxia telangiectasia[†] |
| | Friedreich's ataxia |
| | Amino acid disorders[†] |
| | Spinocerebellar ataxia (esp. SCA 17)[†] |
| Autoimmune (including post-infectious) | Systemic lupus erythematosus (SLE)[*] |
| | Antiphospholipid syndrome[*] |
| | Behçet's syndrome[*] |
| | Coeliac disease[†] |
| | Hashimoto's thyroiditis[*] |
| | Vasculitis[*] |
| | Sydenham's chorea[*] |
| | PANDAS[*] |
| | NMDA receptor antibodies-related |
| | GABA-B receptor antibodies |
| | Paraneoplastic chorea (CRMP5 antibodies) |
| Infections | Human immunodeficiency virus (HIV)[*] |
| | Abscesses in the basal ganglia from any cause[*] |
| | Creutzfeldt–Jakob disease (esp. new variant CJD)[†] |
| Drugs | Dopamine receptor-blocking drugs[†] |
| | Levodopa[†] |
| | Stimulants[*] |
| | Oral contraceptive pill[*] |
| | Anticonvulsants |
| | Anticholinergics, $Ca^{2+}$ antagonists[*] |
| Structural lesions (vascular[*], demyelination[*], tumour[†]) | Lesions of the basal ganglia from any cause (often caudate nucleus) |
| Metabolic | Disorders of thyroid, parathyroid, glucose, sodium, calcium, magnesium[*] |
| | Chorea gravidarum[*] |
| Paroxysmal chorea | Paroxysmal kinesigenic dyskinesia[†] |
| | Paroxysmal non-kinesigenic dyskinesia[†] |
| Other | Post-cardiac bypass (post-pump syndrome)[*] |

[*] Acute onset.
[†] Gradual onset.

# Approach to the patient with chorea

### History
- Age at onset.
- Character of onset—acute or gradual.
- Drug exposure, in particular DRBs. Remember that these drugs are not just used to treat psychiatric illness, but also to treat nausea and vertigo.
- Family history. Beware of 'disappearing' relatives or mysterious deaths—in many families with HD, affected relatives in the past may have committed suicide, been admitted to psychiatric institutions, or simply vanished without a diagnosis being made. Also consider non-paternity.
- Other neurological symptoms: incoordination (WD, HD), sensory disturbance (neuroacanthocytosis).
- Psychiatric/behavioural disturbance.
- Systemic symptoms: recurrent miscarriage, migraine, and thrombosis (systemic lupus erythematosus (SLE), antiphospholipid syndrome (APS)), symptoms of thyroid dysfunction.

### Examination
- Observe the patient at rest with the arms relaxed, with the arms outstretched, and while walking. Chorea may be revealed by a cognitive task, e.g. asking the patient to count backwards from 100 with their eyes closed.
- Note the distribution of chorea (e.g. facial, hemichorea).
- Other neurological signs: other movement disorder (e.g. tics in WD or HD), eye movement disorder (HD), upper motor neuron signs (brain lesion), peripheral neuropathy (neuroacanthocytosis), cerebellar signs (WD, HD), cognitive impairment (HD, WD).
- Systemic signs: rash, arthropathy (SLE), Kayser–Fleischer rings, sunflower cataracts (WD), signs of thyroid disease.

### Investigation
- Choice of investigation is guided by history and examination. Consider the age at onset and the character of onset of the chorea to narrow down the differential diagnosis and investigations needed (Tables 7.1 and 7.2).
- Consider:
  - brain imaging
  - blood testing for autoantibodies (e.g. double-stranded DNA, antiphospholipid), electrolytes, thyroid function, uric acid, and amino acids
  - blood for acanthocytes: a single negative result is not sufficient to fully exclude the presence of acanthocytes (→ p. 170)
  - testing for WD (→ p. 220) and neuroferritinopathy (→ p. 227); genetic testing for HD (→ p. 164) and DRPLA.

### Treatment
- Symptomatic treatment is typically with tetrabenazine or DRBs (→ p. 153).

**Table 7.2** Causes of chorea by typical age at onset

| Onset typically <18 years | |
|---|---|
| Inherited/degenerative disorders | Wilson's disease |
| | Lesch–Nyhan syndrome |
| | Benign hereditary chorea |
| | Ataxia telangiectasia |
| | Amino acid disorders |
| | Friedreich's ataxia |
| Autoimmune (including post-infectious) | Sydenham's chorea |
| | PANDAS |
| Metabolic | Disturbances of glucose |
| Paroxysmal chorea | Paroxysmal kinesigenic dyskinesia |
| | Paroxysmal non-kinesigenic dyskinesia |
| Other | Post-cardiac bypass (post-pump chorea) |
| **Onset typically >18 years** | |
| Inherited/degenerative disorders | Huntington's disease (HD) |
| | HD-like syndromes |
| | Dentatorubropallidoluysian atrophy |
| | Neuroacanthocytosis |
| | McLeod's syndrome |
| | SCA 17 |
| | C9ORF72 mutations (➲ p. 117) |
| | Neuroferritinopathy |
| Autoimmune (including post-infectious) | Systemic lupus erythematosus |
| | Antiphospholipid syndrome |
| | Behçet's syndrome |
| | Hashimoto's thyroiditis |
| | Vasculitis |
| | Coeliac disease |
| Infections | Creutzfeldt–Jakob disease (esp. new variant CJD) |
| Lesions of the basal ganglia | Vascular, demyelinating |
| Metabolic >55–60 years | Disorders of thyroid, parathyroid, glucose, sodium, calcium, magnesium |
| | Polycythaemia rubra vera |
| **Variable age at onset** | |
| Drugs | Anticonvulsants, contraceptive pill, etc. |
| Lesions of the basal ganglia | Tumours, abscesses |
| Other | Chorea gravidarum |

# Huntington's disease

HD is an autosomal dominant degenerative disease characterized by progressive behavioural disturbance, dementia, and movement disorder, usually chorea (see Video 7.2: Huntington's disease). George Huntington was a nineteenth-century GP in North America, who first observed patients with the syndrome that bears his name while following his father, also a GP, on his rounds. The first description was published by Huntington in 1872, although a Norwegian physician Johan Lund had described a similar condition 12 years previously.

## Epidemiology

HD affects approximately 4–8 per 100 000, and males and females equally. There are communities with high prevalence rates, e.g. the population of Moray Firth in Scotland and in Venezuela, in contrast with low rates in Japanese and African Americans.

## Clinical features

- Age at onset is variable but is usually in the fourth decade. Young onset (<18 years) is rare and may present with parkinsonism, rather than chorea (this is called the Westphal variant).
- Onset may be with psychiatric/behavioural disturbance, neurological symptoms, or both.
- Initial psychiatric/behavioural symptoms are typically: lack of inhibition leading to socially inappropriate behaviour, disorganization, apathy, depression, and paranoia. Cognitive function is often initially well preserved.
- Initial neurological symptoms and signs are typically: chorea, tics, gait disturbance, and incoordination.
- Examination usually reveals a combination of generalized chorea and tics. Chorea and tics often affect the face, leading to a rather characteristic pattern of rapidly changing facial expression. There will often be difficulty with maintaining postures, e.g. keeping the tongue protruded.
- The eye movement disorder of HD combines the following:
  - slowed hypometric saccades in younger patients
  - distractibility and impersistence of gaze
  - difficulty in initiating saccades. Patients will often blink or use a thrust of the head in order to shift their gaze from one point to another.
- Gait is often bizarre and more severely affected than one would expect from the degree of chorea.
- Upper motor neuron signs may be present.
- With disease progression, chorea often gives way to more prominent dystonia and parkinsonism.

### Investigations
- Genetic testing is a reliable method of diagnosis and is widely available (➲ p. 166). Brain imaging will often show caudate atrophy.

### Differential diagnosis of Huntington's disease
- **HD-like syndromes**: these are very rare inherited conditions that can have a very similar clinical presentation to HD.
  - HDL-1: a dominantly inherited prion disease due to a 192 base pair insertion in the coding region of the prion protein gene.
  - HDL-2: a dominantly inherited disorder with similar clinical features to HD due to mutations in the junctophillin-3 (*JPH3*) gene. This disorder has only ever been reported in African Americans, with the exception of one family from Brazil with Spanish/Portuguese ancestry. Affected individuals may have acanthocytosis. Recently, families with predominant parkinsonism, rather than chorea, have been reported.
  - HDL-3: an autosomal recessive condition linked to chromosome 4p15.3. Patients present in childhood with an HD-like phenotype. The causative gene is not known.
  - HDL-4: this is the same disorder as SCA 17. This dominantly inherited condition has a very variable presentation and is due to an expanded CAG repeat in the *TBP* gene on chromosome 6.
- **Other dominantly inherited chorea syndromes**:
  - benign hereditary chorea
  - DRPLA is rare in Western countries, but commoner than HD in Japan. Juvenile cases present usually with a myoclonus epilepsy phenotype (➲ p. 187), while adults develop chorea, ataxia, and dementia
  - *C9ORF72* mutations, which most commonly cause FTD-ALS spectrum disorders, have been identified as a cause of HD phenocopies
  - Neuroferritinopathy (➲ p. 227) presents in midlife with chorea or dystonia and other features. Orofacial action-specific dystonia related to speech is characteristic, and iron deposition can be seen on MRI imaging
  - SCA 8, SCA 14.
- **Other non-dominantly inherited chorea syndromes**: WD, neuroacanthocytosis, mitochondrial disease, Friedreich's ataxia, ataxia with oculomotor apraxia (AOA), and ataxia telangiectasia (AT) can sometimes cause confusion with HD. These disorders have typical age at onset in the first two decades of life.
- **Coeliac disease**: can cause chorea and cognitive decline. Usually, however, it causes cerebellar ataxia, peripheral neuropathy, and cortical myoclonus.

# Genetics and genetic counselling in Huntington's disease

## Genetics of Huntington's disease

- HD is a CAG triplet-repeat disorder. A mutation in the *huntingtin* (*HTT*) gene on chromosome 4 causes an enlarged polyglutamine portion to be added to the huntingtin protein, associated with gain-of-function toxicity.
- The exact function of huntingtin in the cell is unknown, but the mutated protein forms aggregates within cells, leading to cell death.
- The number of CAG repeats in the *huntingtin* gene determines whether disease will occur: <35 repeats, no HD; 36–39 repeats, HD may or may not occur; and ≥40 or more repeats, HD will occur.
- As with every other triplet-repeat disorder, HD shows anticipation, e.g. the disease may develop earlier in life in each successive generation.
- Higher repeat numbers are associated with a younger age at onset, but this association is not perfect, and it is not possible to accurately predict the likely age at onset from the repeat length. Juvenile HD is usually (approximately 90% of cases) inherited from the father because of the greater chance of lengthening repeats during spermatogenesis, as opposed to oogenesis.

## Genetic counselling in Huntington's disease

HD is a devastating disease, and a positive diagnosis has genetic implications for other family members. Specialist units for the assessment, counselling, and management of those with HD are not universally available. Therefore, an understanding of the importance of genetic counselling in HD is essential for all those who may be involved in the care of such patients.

### Counselling the patient with symptoms suggestive of Huntington's disease

- Prior to testing, the possibility of HD must be discussed with the patient. There is often insufficient time to do this at the initial consultation, and a further appointment may be needed, with the patient encouraged to bring a family member or friend if they wish.
- The following should be discussed:
  - the nature, course, and prognosis of HD
  - the mode of inheritance and the implications for family members of a positive test
  - the effect of a positive result on mortgage applications, health, and life insurance
  - the possible results: negative, positive, or indeterminate
  - sources of support and reliable information
  - testing is the patient's choice.
- If the patient consents to testing, the probable delay before the test result is available should be explained, and an appropriate follow-up appointment given.

### Counselling at-risk individuals without symptoms
- The diagnosis of HD within a family will often lead family members to seek advice on pre-symptomatic testing. On examination, some will be found to have physical signs of HD, in which case advice is as described in Counselling the patient with symptoms suggestive of Huntington's disease, ➔ p. 164.
- For truly asymptomatic individuals, one should pay more attention to the effects on mortgage, insurance, and the uncertainty that will be caused by an indeterminate test result.

### Other situations
- Pre-implantation and fetal testing for HD is possible but clearly requires extensive counselling, which is best provided by a regional genetics service in conjunction with obstetric services.
- Pre-symptomatic testing of people under the age of 18 is not permitted.
- Testing of minors with symptoms suggestive of HD requires specialist counselling and may be best achieved with a regional genetics service in conjunction with paediatric services.

### Support after test results
- Ideally, a strategy should be in place to provide adequate support for patients and families after the test result.
- Adequate genetic counselling should have produced a good relationship with the patient and family, as well as a patient who is well informed about HD.
- Patient support organizations can be invaluable in providing ongoing support for patients and their families (➔ p. 174).
- Clear routes of access to neurological and psychiatric services should be established to ensure adequate support as needed.

# Management of Huntington's disease

Currently, no treatment has been shown to cure or slow the progression of HD. Management of HD is best achieved within a multidisciplinary team, allowing combined management of neurological, psychiatric, medical, and social issues.

## Psychiatric symptoms

These are often more responsible for disability in HD than the movement disorder. Involvement of psychiatric services is often required. Common treatment approaches include the following:
- SSRIs for depression and anxiety
- benzodiazepines for anxiety and poor sleep
- atypical DRBs for psychosis and hallucinations (may cause movement disorder with chronic use)
- psychological therapies.

## Neurological symptoms

Chorea and tics may be a minor part of the disability caused to the patient by HD. Often family members are more distressed by the abnormal movements than the patient. If treatment is required, options include the following:
- tetrabenazine (→ p. 153)
- DRBs, e.g. sulpiride (→ p. 153)
- other drugs that have been reported to occasionally improve chorea include amantadine and sodium valproate.

## Other symptoms
- Maintenance of weight through a high-calorie diet.
- SLT to assess and treat swallowing difficulty and speech disturbance.
- Early discussion of preferences regarding feeding (PEG insertion) and long-term care is essential.

# Chorea and acanthocytosis

Acanthocytes are red blood cells that have a spiculated (spiky) membrane. A number of neurological disorders are associated with the presence of acanthocytes in the peripheral blood. Three of these (neuroacanthocytosis, McLeod's syndrome, and HD-like 2 (HDL-2)) can present with chorea.

### Testing for acanthocytes
- Abnormalities of red cell shape which can superficially look like acanthocytosis are seen in uraemia, hepatic failure, post-splenectomy, and simply in blood that has been stored for too long or at too high a pH.
- Therefore, accurate identification of acanthocytes needs to be performed by a trained technician provided with fresh blood smears.
- Three negative smears are usually required to be sure that no acanthocytes are present.
- A pathological percentage of acanthocytes in a smear is >3%.

### Neuroacanthocytosis
- An autosomal recessive condition due to mutations in the *VPS13A* gene (formerly called *CHAC*) on chromosome 9q. The gene product is called chorein.
- Affected patients usually present in the third decade with orofacial chorea and dystonia, often with writhing movements of the tongue leading to 'feeding dystonia'. Other signs include tics, parkinsonism, and head banging.
- An axonal neuropathy occurs and may be the presenting feature.
- Progressive generalized chorea, dystonia, and cognitive decline occur. Arrhythmias and cardiomyopathies have been reported in many cases, and cardiac screening and surveillance are important.
- Acanthocytes (often 20–30%) are present. Creatine kinase (CK) is often raised. Brain MRI typically shows caudate and putaminal atrophy. Genetic testing is not widely available. Mutations almost always cause loss of function of the gene, and therefore reduction in the amount of chorein in the cell. Therefore, chorein levels can be assessed in blood cells using Western blotting, as an alternative to genetic testing, but again is not widely available (see Useful websites and addresses, ➔ p. 174). Other causes of acanthocytosis should be sought (Box 7.1).
- Prognosis is variable and is dependent on the development of cardiac and bulbar symptoms. No specific treatment is available.

### McLeod's syndrome
- McLeod's syndrome is an X-linked condition caused by mutations in the *XK* gene. The XK protein is essential for the expression of the Kell group of antigens, the most important group of red cell surface antigens after the A, B, O, and rhesus groups.

- Affected patients are male, and most simply have mild haemolytic anaemia and acanthocytosis. Diagnosis is by demonstrating reduced expression of the Kell antigens on red blood cells.
- Some patients with McLeod's syndrome have peripheral neuropathy or progressive myopathy. Rarely, patients (including one female case) may present with an identical syndrome to neuroacanthocytosis.

### Huntington's disease-like 2 (HDL-2)

- This very rare condition has only been reported in African Americans and is a dominantly inherited disorder with identical symptoms to HD. It is due to mutations in the *junctophillin-3* gene.

> **Box 7.1 Acanthocytosis and neurological disease**
>
> *Acanthocytosis and chorea*
> - Neuroacanthocytosis
> - McLeod's syndrome (rare)
> - HD-like 2 disease (very rare)
>
> *Acanthocytosis and other neurological problems*
> - **Abetalipoproteinaemia**: autosomal recessive fat malabsorption syndrome. Presents in childhood (and rarely in adulthood) with steatorrhoea and failure to thrive. Neurological symptoms (cerebellar syndrome, peripheral neuropathy, pigmentary retinopathy) are caused by secondary vitamin A and E deficiency and are preventable by vitamin supplementation. Serum cholesterol and triglycerides are very low, and lipoprotein electrophoresis reveals the absence of apolipoprotein B.
> - **Hypobetalipoproteinaemia**: an autosomal dominant fat malabsorption syndrome with similar symptoms to abetalipoproteinaemia, but often not as severe. Low-density lipoprotein (LDL) cholesterol is low, and electrophoresis of lipoproteins reveals low levels of apolipoprotein B.
> - **HARP syndrome** (hypoprebetalipoproteinaemia, acanthocytosis, and retinitis pigmentosa): an autosomal recessive condition due to mutations in the pantothenate kinase 2 gene (*PANK2*) and characterized by generalized dystonia (→ p. 224).

# Other causes of chorea

## Autoimmune causes of chorea

### Sydenham's chorea
Thomas Sydenham (1624–1689) was an English physician of great repute, sometimes called 'the English Hippocrates'. He was particularly interested in epidemics, and the Great Plague of London (1665–1666) provided him with ample material. He also valued the powers of first-hand observation of disease, and his writings were published in many editions, even in his lifetime, translated into French and English from the original Latin.

He described chorea affecting children with acute onset and usually resolving after weeks or months. Sydenham's chorea is now recognized as an autoimmune condition triggered by streptococcal infection. It may occur alone or with symptoms and signs of rheumatic fever (carditis, arthritis, rash).

- Patients typically present with acute onset of chorea within days to weeks (but reportedly up to 6 months) following streptococcal infection. Tics and dystonia may also occur and may predominate. Associated behavioural disturbance is common.
- Typical age at onset is late childhood/teens, and females are more commonly affected than males. Rates of Sydenham's chorea in developed countries have dramatically declined with antibiotic use, but recently rates have increased, possibly due to new strains of *Streptococcus*.
- Likely pathophysiology is via 'molecular mimicry' where antibodies formed against *Streptococcus* also bind to the basal ganglia.
- Within 6 months, most patients will experience full remission of symptoms, although 20% will experience a recurrence.
- A small proportion of patients do not recover and have chronic chorea.
- Patients should receive penicillin at onset of symptoms and then take penicillin prophylaxis at least into adulthood to prevent recurrence.
- There are anecdotal reports of successful treatment with IVIG and plasma exchange in refractory cases.
- Chorea in pregnancy (chorea gravidarum) is much commoner in patients with previous Sydenham's chorea.
- PANDAS is a related condition and is discussed in Chapter 6 (➲ p. 156).

### Antiphospholipid syndrome
APS can occur as an isolated condition or in association with SLE. There are circulating antibodies to phospholipids (also known as anti-cardiolipin antibodies). Patients often have a history of recurrent miscarriage, migraine, and thrombosis, and may have additional signs and symptoms suggestive of SLE (e.g. rash, arthritis).

A number of movement disorders have been associated with APS, including chorea, tics, stereotypies, parkinsonism, and myoclonus. The aetiology is thought to be vascular (infarction or 'sluggish' blood flow), and response of symptoms to warfarin or aspirin has been reported.

*Other autoimmune disorders*
Chorea has been reported in patients with NMDA receptor antibodies encephalitis and in patients with antibodies related to an underlying neoplasia (e.g. CRPM5 antibodies). Moreover, chorea has been reported in Behçet's syndrome, polyarteritis nodosa, and primary CNS vasculitis, all probably due to vascular insult to the basal ganglia. Chorea and cognitive decline have been reported in association with coeliac disease, but the pathophysiology is uncertain.

## Structural causes of chorea

Lesions affecting the basal ganglia from any cause (vascular, tumour, abscess, demyelination) can cause chorea. Lesions are usually in the caudate nucleus and commonly cause chorea affecting the opposite side of the body (hemichorea). Lesions of the STN (and the caudate) may cause hemiballismus—wild flinging movements of the limbs. Vascular lesions often cause acute onset of hemichorea/ballism. Tetrabenazine or atypical DRBs can treat symptoms, but, if due to vascular lesions, they often resolve spontaneously.

## Drug-induced chorea

Chorea can be caused by chronic exposure to levodopa in PD, and DRBs (➔ p. 258). Exposure to many other drugs, most importantly the oral contraceptive pill, has been associated with chorea (➔ p. 260). Anticholinergics, often used for the treatment of dystonia or tremor, can also cause chorea.

## Benign hereditary chorea

This is an autosomal dominant condition presenting in infancy with symmetrical distal chorea of the limbs. It is not progressive, and other neurological symptoms and signs do not usually occur. It can be difficult to differentiate from myoclonus dystonia (➔ p. 182). Mutations in the *TITF-1* gene on chromosome 14q have been reported in some families, but testing is not widely available. This gene is involved in function of the thyroid gland and the lung, and some patients with *TITF-1* mutations have a combination of thyroid disease, lung disease, and chorea—'thyroid–brain–lung syndrome'. In some families with *TITF-1* mutations, the phenotype may resemble myoclonus dystonia. ADCY5 mutations may also cause a BHC phenotype (p.311)

## Senile chorea

A syndrome of slowly progressive chorea affecting elderly people has been described. It is unlikely to be a real clinical entity and probably represents a combination of undiagnosed causes of chorea, including HD and vascular lesions.

## Useful websites and addresses

- **Huntington's Disease Association (UK):** Suite 24, Liverpool Science Park, Innovation Centre 1, 131 Mount Pleasant, Liverpool, L3 5TF. Tel: 0151 331 5444; http://www.hda.org.uk. Excellent source of information and support. Has network of regional care advisors who can meet with, and talk to, patients in their area.
- **Huntington's Disease Society of America:** http://www.hdsa.org.
- **Advocacy for Neuroacanthocytosis Patients (UK):** http://www.naadvocacy.org. UK-based charity supporting patients with neuroacanthocytosis.
- **International Parkinson and Movement Disorder Society:** http://www.movementdisorders.org.
- Adrian.Danek@med.uni-muenchen.de Chorein testing available on a research basis.

# Chapter 8

# Myoclonus

Introduction *176*
Approach to the patient with myoclonus *180*
Inherited myoclonic syndromes: 1 *182*
Inherited myoclonic syndromes: 2 *184*
Inherited myoclonic syndromes: 3 *186*
Acquired myoclonus *190*
Treatment of myoclonus *192*
Useful websites and addresses *194*

# CHAPTER 8 **Myoclonus**

# Introduction

### Definition and description
Myoclonus comprises brief electric shock-like jerks. It is a common normal experience. For example, hiccups and jerks of the body when falling asleep (hypnogogic jerks) or on waking (hypnopompic jerks) are forms of myoclonus that are common normal phenomena. Rarely, severe persistent hiccups can occur as part of symptomatic myoclonus (e.g. in liver failure). Similarly, when feeding or while sleeping, infants may have small-amplitude, generalized myoclonic jerks. Affected babies are otherwise entirely normal, and no other symptoms occur. No treatment is needed, and the myoclonus usually resolves within 6–12 months. One should differentiate these normal phenomena from abnormal myoclonus.

#### What causes myoclonus?
Myoclonus is caused by brief activation of one muscle, or more usually a group of muscles, leading to a jerk of the affected body part. This activation can arise from the cortex, subcortical structures (including the brainstem), spinal cord, or nerve roots and plexi. The cerebellum has been recently implicated in the pathophysiology of cortical myoclonus.

Myoclonus is different from tremor where alternate activation of agonists and antagonists produces a shaking movement. Myoclonus is different from dystonia where prolonged simultaneous activation of agonists and antagonists occurs, pulling the affected limb into an abnormal posture.

#### Negative myoclonus
Sometimes myoclonus produces a temporary cessation of muscle activity—negative myoclonus. If negative myoclonus affects the legs, causing the so-called 'bouncy legs syndrome', then the patient may fall. The 'liver flap' (asterixis) that medical students are taught to look for in patients with suspected liver failure is caused by negative myoclonus.

#### Cortical versus subcortical myoclonus
Myoclonus may have a different clinical appearance, depending upon whether it arises from cortical or subcortical areas:
- cortical: typically distal, small-amplitude, often focal; if stimulus-sensitive, often sensitive to touch
- subcortical: typically proximal, large-amplitude, often generalized; if stimulus-sensitive, often sensitive to sound.

### Differential diagnosis of myoclonus
Myoclonus has a huge differential diagnosis. As a result, it is even more important than usual to look for associated symptoms and signs and to pay particular attention to the history. These will often give clues that allow the diagnostic possibilities to be narrowed down considerably. Table 8.1 gives a list of causes of myoclonus, divided under some broad subheadings.

**Table 8.1** Causes of myoclonus

| | |
|---|---|
| Physiological myoclonus | Hypnic jerks, hiccups |
| | Benign infantile myoclonus with feeding/sleep |
| Inherited causes | Myoclonus dystonia (subcortical) |
| | Familial cortical tremor (cortical) |
| | Myoclonus with epilepsy (cortical):<br>• Benign myoclonic epilepsy of infancy<br>• Juvenile myoclonic epilepsy<br>• Early infantile myoclonic encephalopathy<br>• West's syndrome<br>• Lennox–Gastaut syndrome<br>• Familial cortical tremor with epilepsy (FCTME) |
| | Progressive myoclonic epilepsy and ataxia (cortical and/or subcortical):<br>• Lafora body disease<br>• Unverricht–Lundborg disease<br>• Neuronal ceroid lipofuscinosis<br>• Sialidosis<br>• Myoclonus epilepsy with ragged red fibres (MERRF)<br>• Dentatorubropallidoluysian atrophy (DRPLA)<br>• Action myoclonus renal failure syndrome (*SCARB2* mutations) |
| | Genetic Creutzfeldt–Jakob disease (cortical) |
| | Spinocerebellar ataxias |
| Acquired causes | |
| Sporadic neurodegenerative conditions | Plus dementia:<br>• Alzheimer's disease<br>• Dementia with Lewy bodies<br>• Creutzfeldt–Jakob disease<br>• Huntington's disease |
| | Plus parkinsonism:<br>• Corticobasal degeneration<br>• Multiple system atrophy (polyminimyoclonus) |

(Continued)

### Table 8.1 (Contd.)

| | |
|---|---|
| Systemic/drug-related/lesions | Liver failure (negative myoclonus) |
| | Renal failure |
| | Drug intoxication (alcohol, lithium, carbamazepine) |
| | Toxins (lead poisoning) |
| | Post-hypoxia (Lance–Adams syndrome) |
| | Spinal cord/root/plexus injury (focal/segmental) |
| | Palatal myoclonus (Guillain–Mollaret triangle lesion) |
| Infections | Whipple's disease |
| | Subacute sclerosing panencephalitis (SSPE) |
| Autoimmune | Progressive encephalomyelitis with rigidity and myoclonus |
| | Coeliac disease (cortical myoclonus) |
| | Paraneoplastic (opsoclonus–myoclonus syndrome) |

INTRODUCTION 179

# Approach to the patient with myoclonus

## History
- Age at onset.
- Character of onset (acute, gradual).
- Precipitating factors at onset (hypoxia, encephalitis, drug use, metabolic disturbance, brain/cord/plexus injury).
- Is the myoclonus alcohol-responsive?
- Take a thorough drug history.
- Family history (if positive, note mode of inheritance—autosomal dominant, recessive, maternal, or paternal).
- Associated symptoms—especially epilepsy, ataxia, cognitive decline.
- Static or progressive symptoms?

## Examination
- Look for myoclonus at rest, on posture of the arms, and during action.
- Note distribution of myoclonus (generalized/segmental/focal).
- Note amplitude of jerks.
- Are the jerks rhythmic?
- Look for stimulus sensitivity. Ask the patient to stretch out their arms in front of them and close their eyes. Gently flick their outstretched fingers, and see if this triggers myoclonic jerks. With the patient in the same position, clap your hands loudly to look for auditory triggering of myoclonus.
- Look for negative myoclonus, e.g. 'bouncy legs' (giving way of the legs while standing/walking), asterixis.
- Examine for other neurological signs, especially cerebellar signs, retinopathy.
- Examine for signs of systemic disease (e.g. liver failure).

## Investigation
- Given the extensive differential diagnosis of myoclonus, numerous investigations are possible, and many are invasive and expensive. Therefore, it is important to use the associated clinical features present with the myoclonus to narrow the differential, and hence the number of tests needed.
- Electrophysiological tests can be very helpful to characterize the disorder. Examples are given on ➔ p. 181.

## Treatment
- Symptomatic treatment is available for myoclonus. It is often necessary to use a combination of drugs to treat myoclonus. Most drugs for myoclonus cause sedation as a main side effect, and this often limits treatment efficacy.
- Treatments for myoclonus are discussed in detail on ➔ p. 192.

## Electrophysiological investigations in myoclonus

### Electromyography to record jerks
Myoclonic jerks are typically caused by very brief (<50 ms) bursts of muscle activity. It is not possible to consistently voluntarily produce EMG bursts of less than about 50–75 ms, and therefore this is strong evidence of organicity. However, some organic myoclonus syndromes cause bursts of muscle activity lasting longer than 75 ms.

### 'Back-averaging' of jerks
In cortical myoclonus, jerks will be preceded by a cortical discharge, which can be recorded on electroencephalography (EEG). A single discharge will be impossible to pick out amongst the background EEG activity. Therefore, EEG is performed during EMG recording of a number of jerks. The EEG trace shortly before each jerk is then selected and averaged, and this will have the effect of revealing any underlying cortical discharge.

### Pre-movement electroencephalographic potentials
Prior to normal voluntary movement, a slow-rising wave called the *bereitschafts* potential (BP) is seen on the EEG. If psychogenic myoclonus is suspected, averaged recording of EEG just prior to jerks, as detailed in 'Back-averaging of jerks' above, can be helpful, as a BP is often seen if the cause of the jerks is psychogenic.

### Somatosensory evoked potentials
In cortical myoclonus, very large responses may be recorded from the somatosensory cortex when somatosensory evoked potentials (SSEPs) are tested. These are known as giant SSEPs.

## Inherited myoclonic syndromes: 1

### Myoclonus dystonia
- Typical age at onset is in infancy/early childhood. However, symptoms may be mild and therefore not noticed at onset (📽 see Video 8.1: Myoclonus dystonia).
- Typical clinical features are very brief myoclonic jerks, mainly affecting the neck and arms. Jerks are so brief that they have been described as 'lightning jerks' or 'tic-tac' jerks.
- Dystonia may be present but tends to be a minor feature, compared with the myoclonus. If present, dystonia mainly affects the neck and arms.
- Myoclonus and dystonia are often very responsive to alcohol.
- Some patients may have additional psychiatric disturbances such as obsessive–compulsive behaviour, anxiety, and depression.
- Autosomal dominant inheritance is common.
- A proportion of patients (around 30%) have mutations in the epsilon sarcoglycan gene on chromosome 7q (DYT11). This gene shows 'maternal imprinting', meaning that children inheriting the mutation from their mothers almost never develop symptoms. Genetic testing is available in a small number of centres.
- Other genes have been found to cause myoclonus dystonia that typically cause other phenotypes such as mutations in the *TITF-1* gene causing benign hereditary chorea (➔ p. 173) and *ANO3* (DYT24) typically causing adult-onset tremulous segmental dystonia (➔ p. 202)
- A new locus has been identified for myoclonus dystonia (DYT15), but no gene has been identified yet.
- Myoclonus is electrophysiologically of the subcortical type (i.e. no EEG abnormalities, no giant SSEPs).
- Treatment is symptomatic (➔ p. 192), and the need for psychiatric evaluation and treatment should be considered.

### Familial cortical tremor with or without epilepsy

This is a syndrome of autosomal dominant myoclonus which presents with very fine distal limb myoclonus (often described as 'shivering' of the fingers) that superficially resembles ET. However, EMG shows discrete bursts of muscle activity, rather than the oscillating agonist–antagonist activity seen in tremor, and giant SSEPs occur.
- Variable age at onset (10–50 years).
- Two loci have been identified (FCTME1 and 2), but as yet no genes.
- Generalized seizures and cerebellar signs may occur.
- Responds to sodium valproate, primidone, and benzodiazepines.

# Inherited myoclonic syndromes: 2

## Myoclonus and epilepsy
Some myoclonus syndromes occur in combination with epilepsy. There is a specific group of myoclonus syndromes associated with epilepsy and ataxia (progressive myoclonic epilepsy–ataxia syndromes (PMEA)), and these are considered separately (➔ p. 186).

### Myoclonus and epilepsy without encephalopathy
- Benign myoclonic epilepsy of infancy: presents in children under the age of 2 years. Myoclonic seizures occur, and 3 Hz spike-and-wave discharges are seen on EEG. Sodium valproate is often effective.
- Juvenile myoclonic epilepsy: onset in teenage years of myoclonic jerks and generalized seizures. Typical precipitants of myoclonic jerks and seizures are alcohol use and sleep deprivation. Symptoms tend to be most marked in the mornings; patients will often report episodes where they have dropped their morning cup of tea because of a myoclonic jerk—'tea-cup epilepsy'. EEG shows a characteristic 3–5 Hz polyspike and wave pattern. Sodium valproate and lamotrigine are effective.
- Epilepsia partialis continua (EPC): rhythmic jerking of a limb may occur secondary to constant epileptic discharges from the motor cortex. The cause is often a lesion (tumour, infarct, dysgenesis), and the EEG will show focal spiking from the relevant motor cortex.

### Myoclonus and epilepsy with encephalopathy
A number of myoclonic epilepsy syndromes are associated with encephalopathy. These are typically of infantile onset and have numerous causes, including cortical malformations, metabolic disorders, and perinatal injury. These syndromes include the following.
- Early infantile myoclonic encephalopathy—Ohtahara syndrome: this comprises myoclonic seizures beginning before 3 months of age, with progressive encephalopathy.
- West's syndrome: infantile spasms (jackknife convulsions), developmental arrest, and hypsarrhythmia on EEG (diffuse, disorganized high-voltage slow waves, spikes, and sharp waves during wakefulness) occurring before 1 year of age.
- Lennox–Gastaut syndrome: several seizure types, including myoclonic seizures, characteristic EEG (slow background with 1.5–2.5 Hz slow spike-and-wave discharge), and cognitive decline occurring between 1 and 7 years of age.

# Inherited myoclonic syndromes: 3

## Progressive myoclonic epilepsy–ataxia syndromes

This is a group of rare, but important, conditions which cause progressive myoclonus, epilepsy, and ataxia. Epilepsy may be a minor part of the clinical picture, and progressive ataxia and myoclonus may predominate. This phenotype is also called Ramsay–Hunt syndrome. Age at onset, prognosis, and diagnostic tests for PMEA are given in Table 8.2.

### Unverricht–Lundborg disease (Baltic myoclonus)

- Autosomal recessive condition with generalized seizures, limb myoclonus, and progressive cerebellar signs. Age at onset is 10–15. Cognitive decline occurs late and is mild. Life expectancy is 50–60 years of age (see Video 8.2: Progressive myoclonic ataxia).
- The cause is a dodecamer-repeat expansion in the cystatin B (*EPM1*, *CSTB*) gene. Genetic testing is widely available.
- Treatment is symptomatic. There are anecdotal reports of dramatic response to *N*-acetylcysteine.

### Lafora body disease

- Autosomal recessive condition characterized by onset of seizures (often occipital) at age 10–15 years, followed by progressive myoclonus, ataxia, and cognitive decline. Death occurs within 2–10 years.
- Lafora bodies are inclusion bodies composed of insoluble carbohydrate. They are found in the brain, muscle, and skin. Skin biopsy is diagnostic.
- A number of different mutations in *NHLRC1* (*EPM2A*) gene have been identified in Lafora body disease, but testing is only on a research basis.

### Neuronal ceroid lipofuscinoses

- Autosomal recessive lysosomal storage disorders with infantile, late-infantile, childhood, and adult-onset forms. The adult-onset form is called Kufs. Collectively, neuronal ceroid lipofuscinoses (NCL) is known as Batten's disease.
- Clinical features: progressive myoclonus, epilepsy, ataxia, spasticity. Parkinsonism can be part of the clinical picture. Retinal degeneration and optic atrophy occur in childhood-onset NCL.
- Inclusion bodies containing the lipopigments ceroid and lipofuscin are seen in eccrine sweat glands (e.g. from an axillary skin biopsy).
- Prognosis is worse in young-onset cases (death within 5–10 years).
- A number of genes have been identified (*CLN1–10*).
- *CLN6* seems to be commoner in adults and adolescents (Kufs disease).

### Sialidosis
- Autosomal recessive disorder of glycoprotein metabolism due to neuraminidase deficiency.
- Type I sialidosis has onset in adolescence, and type II has onset at birth or in infancy. In both, the main clinical features are seizures, myoclonus, ataxia, and a retinal abnormality called a cherry red spot.
- Diagnosis is via measurement of neuraminidase in cultured fibroblasts. Urinary oligosaccharide excretion is elevated.
- Type I is compatible with normal lifespan. Type II causes cognitive decline and death in childhood/teens.
- Mutations in neuraminidase-1 (*NEU1*) gene have been identified as causative.

### Myoclonic epilepsy with ragged red fibres
- Myoclonic epilepsy with ragged red fibres (MERRF) is a disorder of mitochondrial function that causes a variable combination of ataxia, seizures, dementia, spasticity, and muscle weakness.
- Age at onset is typically in late childhood and adolescence but is variable. Maternal inheritance is seen.
- The *A8344G* mutation in mitochondrial DNA is most commonly associated with MERRF, but other mutations are seen. Muscle biopsy is used for diagnosis and shows characteristic 'ragged red fibres'.

### Dentatorubropallidoluysian atrophy
- DRPLA is a dominantly inherited triplet-repeat disorder affecting the *DRPLA* gene on chromosome 12p. The prevalence in Japan is significantly higher than that in Europe and North America.
- May present in childhood or teenage years with progressive dementia, seizures, myoclonus, and ataxia. In adult-onset DRPLA, ataxia, chorea, and cognitive decline are the main clinical features.
- MRI shows degeneration in the areas of the brain suggested by the name of the condition: the dentate and red nuclei, pallidum, and STN. Gene testing is commercially available.
- Haw River syndrome is a syndrome of progressive ataxia without myoclonus or epilepsy described in an African American family who carry the same triplet-repeat expansion as *DRPLA* and who have basal ganglia calcification and signs of demyelination on brain imaging.

### Action myoclonus renal failure syndrome
- Another seemingly rare cause of PMEA without dementia is action myoclonus renal failure syndrome (AMRF).
- Initially described in French Canadians, but has been reported in patients with various ethnic backgrounds.
- Due to mutations in the gene coding for the lysosomal protein SCARB2.
- The distinguishing feature is the occurrence of renal failure due to focal glomerulosclerosis, which, however, may be absent.
- Typical age of onset is around 20 years old, and typically neurological and renal symptoms develop simultaneously in one-third of patients, and renal symptoms are first in one-third.

*'North Sea' progressive myoclonus epilepsy: GOSR2 mutations*
- The cases initially described come from regions bounding the North Sea, extending to the coastal region of northern Norway; patients from northern Netherlands have also been described.
- Homozygous mutations in the Golgi SNAP receptor complex 2 gene (*GOSR2*) have been identified as causative.
- Clinical presentation is characterized by early-onset ataxia (average 2 years of age), followed by myoclonic seizures at the average age of 6.5 years.
- Patients develop multiple seizure types, including generalized tonic–clonic seizures, absence seizures, and drop attacks.
- Scoliosis is almost always present by adolescence, and additional skeletal deformities may be present, including pes cavus and syndactyly. Areflexia is also common.
- Investigations may show elevated serum CK levels, but normal muscle biopsies.
- EMG reveals signs of sensory neuronopathy or anterior horn cell involvement, or both, in patients with absent reflexes.
- The course is progressive, and most patients are wheelchair-bound by adolescence.

Table 8.2 Age at onset, prognosis, and diagnostic tests for progressive myoclonic epilepsy–ataxia syndromes

| Name | Age at onset | Prognosis | Investigation |
|---|---|---|---|
| Lafora body disease | 10–15 years | Death 2–10 years from onset | Lafora bodies in skin biopsy |
| Unverricht–Lundborg disease | 10–15 years | Survival common to fifth to sixth decade | Gene test for repeat expansion in cystatin B gene |
| Neuronal ceroid lipofuscinoses | Variable | In adult-onset form, typically 10–15 years from onset | Axillary skin biopsy shows inclusion bodies in eccrine sweat glands |
| Sialidosis | Type I in teens, type II at birth or in infancy | Type I compatible with normal life expectancy; type II die in childhood | Elevated urinary oligosaccharide excretion; skin biopsy may show vacuolar structures bound to cell membrane |
| MERRF | Variable | Variable, can be normal | Ragged red fibres on muscle biopsy |
| DRPLA | Variable, from childhood to sixth decade | Variable, younger onset associated with more rapid decline | Gene test for triplet repeat expansion in *DRPLA* gene; >48 repeats are pathological |
| AMRF | Around 20 years typically | Variable, younger onset associated with more rapid decline | Gene test available |

# Acquired myoclonus

### Generalized myoclonus with encephalopathy
Generalized myoclonus associated with encephalopathy is commonly caused by metabolic disturbance (e.g. liver failure, renal failure) and drug toxicity.

*Post-hypoxic myoclonus (Lance–Adams syndrome)*
Patients who have a hypoxic insult (e.g. following respiratory arrest, much more commonly than cardiac arrest) can develop a syndrome of non-progressive generalized myoclonus, seizures, ataxia, and a variable degree of encephalopathy (see Video 8.3: Post-hypoxic myoclonus). Mobility is often severely impaired by a combination of positive and negative myoclonus ('bouncy legs') and ataxia. Treatment is symptomatic (p. 192). Cerebrospinal fluid (CSF) serotonin is low in some patients, and there have been anecdotal reports of successful treatment with the serotonergic drug L-5 hydroxytryptophan. No controlled trials are available, and the drug has limited availability and prominent gastrointestinal side effects.

### Focal/segmental myoclonus
*Spinal segmental myoclonus*
Focal lesions affecting the spinal cord (e.g. following trauma, demyelination, or tumour) can produce myoclonus. The myoclonus in this case tends to be confined to muscles innervated by the spinal segments adjacent to the lesion, giving rise to the description 'spinal segmental myoclonus'. Jerking is usually continuous and rhythmical and tends not to be stimulus- or position-sensitive.

Myoclonus is sometimes seen following nerve root or plexus damage, e.g. following radiotherapy for carcinoma of the breast. BT can be helpful in such cases.

*Propriospinal myoclonus*
This is a syndrome of myoclonus affecting the abdominal muscles which causes the trunk to flex suddenly (or rarely extend). This type of myoclonus is typically position-sensitive and worsens, or may only occur when the patient is lying flat. The cause is thought to be within the spinal cord, with an abnormal impulse conducted through slow propriospinal pathways. A spinal cord lesion may be found, and EMG shows muscle activity propagating slowly rostrally and caudally, affecting the abdominal muscles first. A form of propriospinal myoclonus is also described at sleep–wake transition. In many cases, however, propriospinal myoclonus has been thought to be functional (psychogenic).

### Reticular reflex myoclonus
Brainstem lesions can give rise to myoclonus. The myoclonus tends to be stimulus-sensitive, typically to sound. EMG will show myoclonus occurring at very short latency from the provoking stimulus. The spread of myoclonus often starts in the muscles of the shoulder and lower face, spreading up to the orbicularis oculi and down to the limb muscles.

## Generalized myoclonus in sporadic neurodegenerative conditions

### With dementia

Myoclonus is commonly seen in patients with Alzheimer's disease and DLB. Creutzfeldt–Jakob disease (CJD), both classic and new variant forms, can cause myoclonus, and this can be the presenting feature of the condition.

### With parkinsonism

Both CBD (➔ p. 108) and MSA (➔ p. 102) are commonly associated with stimulus-sensitive myoclonus (see Video 8.4: MSA myoclonus). As with other symptoms in CBD, myoclonus often affects only one limb at onset and may then progress to involve other limbs.

## Other conditions

Paraneoplastic syndromes may cause myoclonus. The commonest of these is opsoclonus–myoclonus where jerks affecting the eyes and limbs occur. In children, this is usually secondary to a neuroblastoma.

Coeliac disease has been associated with a number of movement disorders, including myoclonus. This may be generalized but can also affect just a single limb. Gastrointestinal signs of coeliac disease may be absent. Positive anti-gliadin antibodies are usually present, and a small bowel biopsy is diagnostic. A gluten-free diet has been reported to improve movement disorders associated with coeliac disease.

Subacute sclerosing panencephalitis (SSPE), due to reactivation of the measles virus, can cause a syndrome of progressive encephalopathy, typically with periodic 'hung-up' myoclonic jerks, associated with an abnormal EEG. Progressive cognitive and neurological decline is the norm, with death in the majority of patients within 1–2 years. Treatment with inosine pranobex and interferon alfa has been reported anecdotally to be effective, but no controlled data are available.

Progressive encephalomyelitis with rigidity and myoclonus (PERM) is described in detail in Chapter 16.

# Treatment of myoclonus

A number of drugs may be helpful in the symptomatic treatment of myoclonus. Combinations of these drugs are often needed to provide adequate symptom control, but side effects (mainly sedation) can be problematic. We often start with valproate, then add in clonazepam, and then piracetam/levetiracetam, as required or tolerated. BT provides an alternative treatment for those with focal myoclonus. Phenytoin may worsen myoclonus and should be avoided.

### Clonazepam
- Available in 500 micrograms (beige) or 2 mg (white) tablets. Tablets are scored twice.
- Starting dose is 250 micrograms once daily (125 micrograms in the elderly).
- Increase every week by 250 micrograms to reach 500 micrograms to 1 mg bd or tds.
- Maximum dose 8–10 mg daily.
- Main side effects are sedation, depression, and fatigue.

### Primidone
- Available in 250 mg tablets (scored twice).
- Starting dose is 62.5 mg once daily.
- Increase by 62.5 mg every week to reach 250 mg bd or tds, if required or tolerated.
- Maximum dose 1.5 g daily.*
- Main side effects are sedation, ataxia, nausea, and rash. Elderly patients are very susceptible to side effects. Reduce dose very slowly when withdrawing after chronic administration.

### Piracetam
- Available in 800 mg tablets (scored) and oral solution (333.3 mg/mL).
- Starting dose is 1600 mg tds.
- Increase by 1600 mg every week to reach 3200–4800 mg tds.
- Maximum dose 20 g daily
- Main side effects are sedation, diarrhoea, weight gain, and depression.

### Levetiracetam
- Available in 250 mg (blue), 500 mg (yellow), and 1000 mg (white) tablets.
- Starting dose is 250 mg bd, increasing by 250 mg every week to reach 1000 mg bd. Maximum dose 3000 mg daily.
- Main side effects are fatigue, nausea, mood disturbance, and dizziness.

### Sodium valproate
- Available generic 100 mg, 200 mg, and 500 mg tablets, modified-release tablets, granules, modified-release capsules, and oral liquid 200 mg/5 mL (see *British National Formulary* (*BNF*) for full list of formulations).
- Starting dose is 200 mg once daily.
- Increase by 200 mg every 2 weeks to reach 400 mg tds of standard preparations or 600 mg bd of modified-release preparations.
- Maximum dose 2.5 g daily.
- Main side effects include sedation, weight gain, hair thinning, and nausea. Sodium valproate is associated with fetal malformations, and women of childbearing age should be specifically counselled regarding this.

## Useful website
- International Parkinson and Movement Disorder Society: http://www.movementdisorders.org.

# Chapter 9

# Dystonia

Introduction *196*
Approach to the patient with dystonia *200*
Genetic classification of dystonia *202*
Isolated dystonias: 1 *204*
Isolated dystonias: 2 *206*
Isolated dystonias: 3 *208*
Combined dystonias: 1 *210*
Combined dystonias: 2 *214*
Combined dystonias: 3 *218*
Wilson's disease *220*
Treatment of Wilson's disease *222*
Neuronal brain iron accumulation syndromes *224*
Acquired dystonia *230*
Status dystonicus *232*
Treatment of dystonia: strategies *234*
Treatment of dystonia: medical *236*
Treatment of dystonia: botulinum toxin 1 *238*
Treatment of dystonia: botulinum toxin 2 *240*
Treatment of dystonia: botulinum toxin 3 *242*
Treatment of dystonia: surgical *244*
Treatment of dystonia: physical and 'retraining' therapies *246*
Useful websites and addresses *248*

# Introduction

## Definition
Dystonia is defined as involuntary muscle spasm which leads to sustained abnormal postures of the affected body part. Typically, the abnormal postures are not fixed, and slow writhing movements can occur (athetosis) where the dominant muscle activity switches from agonist to antagonist and back again. Tremor commonly occurs with dystonia and tends to affect the same body part. Dystonic tremor is typically jerky, variable in amplitude, and worsened by particular positions of the affected limb and/or the task being undertaken.

## Is it dystonia?
Dystonia has a very variable clinical presentation. In general, dystonia is:
- mobile, rather than fixed
- task- or position-specific
- caused by co-contraction of agonist and antagonist muscles. This can be felt, or detected by EMG
- often improved by a sensory trick or *geste antagoniste*. Often a patient with dystonia will be able to improve the abnormal posture by touching (or even thinking about touching) the body part affected.

## Ways of classifying dystonia
There have been many classification systems over the years. The most commonly used are:

### By distribution
Dystonia can be classified by the distribution of body parts it affects.
- Focal dystonia: one body part only (e.g. hand).
- Segmental: two or more contiguous body parts (e.g. arm and neck).
- Multifocal: two or more non-contiguous body parts (e.g. right arm and left leg).
- Hemidystonia: dystonia affecting one side of the body.
- Generalized: two or more contiguous body parts plus trunk.

### By age at onset
It can be useful to divide patients with dystonia into those with young onset (<25 years) and those with adult onset (>25 years).

### By aetiology
- **Primary dystonia**: dystonia tremor is the only symptom and sign; there is no secondary cause and no neurodegeneration.
- **Dystonia-plus syndromes**: other signs may occur with the dystonia, but there is no secondary cause and no neurodegeneration.
- **Secondary dystonia**: clear secondary cause is present (e.g. brain injury, drug exposure). Dystonia is present with other symptoms and signs.
- **Heredo-degenerative dystonia**: dystonia is present as part of a wider neurodegenerative syndrome.

- **Paroxysmal dystonia**: episodic attacks of dystonia, often no clinical signs between attacks (see ➔ Chapter 11).
- **Psychogenic dystonia**: often fixed postures, with other signs suggesting a psychogenic movement disorder (see ➔ Chapter 15).

## New consensus for classifying dystonia

A new classification of dystonia has been proposed recently along two axes, with axis 1 detailing clinical characteristics and axis 2 detailing the aetiology. One of the biggest changes is that the terms primary and secondary dystonia have been abandoned, replaced by isolated (dystonia with no other signs) and combined (dystonia with other signs).

Axis 1 includes clinical characteristics:
- age of onset (infancy, birth to 2 years; childhood, 3–12 years; adolescence, 13–20 years; early adulthood, 21–40 years; late adulthood, >40 years)
- body distribution (focal, segmental, multifocal, generalized, hemidystonia)
- temporal pattern (disease course: static, progressive; variability: persistent, action-specific, diurnal, paroxysmal)
- associated features (isolated dystonia or combined with another movement disorder—isolated or combined; and occurrence of other neurological or systemic manifestations).

Axis 2 includes the aetiology (Table 9.1):
- nervous system pathology (evidence of degeneration, evidence of structural lesions, or no evidence of degeneration or structural lesions)
- inherited or acquired (inherited: autosomal dominant, autosomal recessive, X-linked recessive, mitochondrial; acquired: perinatal brain injury, infection, drugs, toxic, vascular, neoplastic, brain injury, psychogenic)
- idiopathic (sporadic or familial).

## CHAPTER 9 **Dystonia**

**Table 9.1** Some causes of dystonia

| | |
|---|---|
| Isolated dystonias (former primary) | Young-onset: usually generalized, also called primary torsion dystonia or Oppenheim's dystonia, and often due to *TOR1A* gene mutations (DYT1) <br> Adult onset: <br> Task-specific (e.g. writer's cramp, musician's dystonia) <br> Focal (e.g. oromandibular, torticollis, blepharospasm, dystonic tremor) <br> Rare genetic primary dystonias (e.g. DYT6, GNAL, ANO3) |
| Combined dystonias <br> Inherited | Myoclonus dystonia (due to epsilon sarcoglycan gene mutations or others) <br> Tyrosine hydroxylase deficiency (*TH*) <br> Benign hereditary chorea (*TITF-1* gene mutations) <br> *GTPCH1* mutations carriers (classic dopa-responsive dystonia) <br> Ataxia telangiectasia (*ATM* gene mutations) <br> X-linked dystonia parkinsonism (Lubag) <br> Rapid-onset dystonia parkinsonism (RODP) <br> Neuronal brain iron accumulation syndrome (NBIA) <br> Huntington's disease <br> Wilson's disease <br> Spinocerebellar ataxias <br> Dentatorubropallidoluysian atrophy (DRPLA) <br> Neuroacanthocytosis <br> Mohr–Tranebjaerg syndrome (deafness–dystonia) <br> Metachromatic leukodystrophy <br> GM1/GM2 gangliosidosis <br> Amino acidaemias <br> Niemann–Pick type C |
| Acquired | Brain injury (often putamen) <br> Drugs: many drugs can cause acute dystonia; dopamine receptor-blocking drugs may cause acute and delayed (tardive) dystonia <br> Post-encephalitis |
| Idiopathic | Parkinson's disease <br> Corticobasal degeneration <br> Progressive supranuclear palsy <br> Multiple system atrophy |
| Paroxysmal dystonia | Paroxysmal kinesigenic dyskinesia <br> Paroxysmal non-kinesigenic dyskinesia <br> Paroxysmal exercise-induced dystonia |
| Functional (psychogenic) dystonia | |

# INTRODUCTION

# Approach to the patient with dystonia

## General considerations

### Does the patient have isolated or combined dystonia?
This is the most important clinical question, when faced with a patient with dystonia, and will guide the diagnostic approach. The presence of other signs will give clues for the possible underlying aetiology. Moreover, there are various 'red flags' which suggest that the dystonia may be due to an acquired aetiology or due to a neurodegenerative condition, inherited or otherwise.

- Abnormal birth/perinatal history.
- Developmental delay.
- Previous exposure to drugs (e.g. DRBs).
- Continued progression of symptoms.
- Prominent bulbar involvement by dystonia.
- Unusual distribution of dystonia, given age at onset (Table 9.2).
- Unusual nature of dystonia (e.g. fixed dystonic postures).
- Hemidystonia.

Isolated dystonias have an anatomical distribution, which depends on age at onset. If patients present with an unusual pattern of dystonia for their age at onset, such as leg dystonia in an adult, this is a further clue to an acquired/degenerative cause.

### Differential diagnosis of combined dystonias
There are many causes of combined dystonias, and investigation can be invasive and time-consuming. A useful way to approach the differential diagnosis is to look for other clinical signs that are present with the dystonia. These 'syndromic associations' (e.g. dystonia and peripheral neuropathy or dystonia and parkinsonism) can be very helpful in narrowing down the diagnostic possibilities.

Table 9.2 Distribution of isolated dystonias by age at onset

| Age at onset | Childhood/adolescence | Early adulthood | Late adulthood |
|---|---|---|---|
| Anatomical distribution | GENERALIZED | FOCAL | FOCAL |
| | Typically limb onset, spares head and neck | Task-specific upper limb dystonia (e.g. writer's cramp) | Head and neck, dystonia affecting legs almost never seen |

# Important points to remember on history and examination

## History
- Age at onset.
- Nature of onset (acute or gradual).
- Course of symptoms (static, progressive then plateau, progressive).
- Body part(s) affected.
- Task/position specificity.
- Any precipitating factor(s)—in particular brain injury, drug exposure, and excessive practice of particular movement (e.g. musicians).
- Any sensory tricks that can improve symptoms.
- Any other relieving factors? For example, some patients with leg dystonia may report that they are better when they walk backwards or run than when they try to walk normally.
- Any family history (remember that some hereditary dystonias are partially penetrant, e.g. DYT1 dystonia and DRD; ➔ p. 204 and ➔ p. 210).
- Any change in symptoms during the course of the day (seen in DRD; ➔ p. 210).
- Birth/perinatal history.
- Developmental history.
- Other neurological symptoms (e.g. seizures, cognitive decline, visual disturbance, incoordination, slowness of movement, stiffness).
- Any systemic symptoms.

## Examination
- Observe the patient at rest with arms outstretched and in 'wing-beating' position, and during slow pronation/supination of the arms, looking for abnormal posture and tremor.
- Examine the patient while walking (ideally with shoes and trousers off/rolled up) to look for abnormal posture of the feet/legs.
- Observe the patient writing—look for abnormal posture of the writing hand, abnormally hard pressure on the paper, overflow with elevation of the elbow/shoulder, and any abnormal movements of the hand not writing (mirror movements).
- Examine for other neurological signs, especially parkinsonism, myoclonus, pyramidal signs, retinopathy, eye movement disorder, neuropathy.
- Examine for systemic signs (e.g. organomegaly).

## Investigation and treatment
This is entirely dependent on the history and examination findings, and is discussed in subsequent sections relating to different types of dystonia.

# Genetic classification of dystonia

A number of genetic causes of dystonia have been designated with DYT numbers—currently DYT1–DYT25 (Table 9.3). This classification system is of limited clinical use for the following reasons.
- It is not an exhaustive list of all genetic causes of dystonia.
- It mixes different phenomenologies and aetiologies of dystonia.
- It contains many conditions that do not have identified gene mutations (some DYT conditions are areas of linkage only) or simply clinical descriptions without genetic information.

Table 9.3 DYT classification of dystonia

| DYT number and name of condition | | Clinical features | Gene | Testing available? |
|---|---|---|---|---|
| DYT1 | AD | Young-onset isolated generalized dystonia | TOR1A | Yes |
| DYT2 | AR | Recessive young-onset isolated dystonia in Spanish gypsy family | ? | No |
| DYT3<br>X-linked dystonia parkinsonism | XR | Dystonia parkinsonism in Filipino males | TAF1 | Yes, on research basis |
| DYT4<br>Whispering dysphonia | AD | Laryngeal dystonia limb dystonia in Australian family | TUBB4A | No |
| DYT5a<br>Dopa-responsive dystonia | AD | Young-onset dystonia parkinsonism responsive to levodopa | GTPCH1 | Yes |
| DYT6 | AD | Adolescent-onset isolated from focal cranio-cervical and limb to generalized dystonia | THAP1 | No |
| DYT7 | AD | German family with isolated cranio-cervical dystonia | Linkage to 18p | No |
| DYT8<br>PNKD | AD | Attacks of dystonia and chorea precipitated by coffee, alcohol, and fatigue | MR1 | Yes, on research basis |
| DYT9<br>(identical to DYT18) | AD | Episodic chorea and ataxia with progressive interictal spasticity | SLC2A1 | No |
| DYT10<br>PKD | AD | Episodes of chorea and dystonia precipitated by sudden movement | PRRT2 | No |

(Continued)

**Table 9.3** (Contd.)

| DYT number and name of condition | | Clinical features | Gene | Testing available? |
|---|---|---|---|---|
| DYT11<br>Myoclonus dystonia | AD | Myoclonus and dystonia | Epsilon sarcoglycan gene | Yes |
| DYT12<br>Rapid-onset dystonia parkinsonism | AD | Acute onset of dystonia following infection/exercise | ATP1A3 | Yes, on research basis |
| DYT13 | AD | Italian family with isolated cranio-cervical dystonia | Linkage to 1p36.13–36.32 | No |
| DYT14<br>(identical to DYT5a) | AD | Dopa-responsive dystonia parkinsonism | GTPCH1 gene | No |
| DYT15<br>Myoclonus dystonia | AD | Myoclonus and dystonia | Linkage to 18p11 | No |
| DYT16 | AR | Young-onset dystonia parkinsonism | PRKRA | Yes, on research basis |
| DYT17 | AR | Autosomal recessive dystonia | Unknown | No |
| DYT18 | AD | Paroxysmal exercise-induced dyskinesia | SLC2A1 | Yes |
| DYT19 | AD | Episodic kinesigenic dyskinesia 2 | Unknown | No |
| DYT20 | AD | Paroxysmal non-kinesigenic dyskinesia 2 | Unknown | No |
| DYT21 | AD | Late-onset pure dystonia | Unknown | No |
| DYT22 | Not listed | | | |
| DYT23 | AD | Adult-onset cranio-cervical dystonia | CIZ1 | No |
| DYT24 | AD | Adult-onset cranio-cervical dystonia | ANO3 | Yes on research basis |
| DYT25 | AD | Adult-onset cranio-cervical dystonia | GNAL | Yes |

AD, autosomal dominant; AR, autosomal recessive; GTPCH1, guanosine triphosphate cyclohydrolase 1; PKD, paroxysmal kinesigenic dyskinesia; PNKD, paroxysmal non-kinesigenic dyskinesia; XR, X-linked recessive.

# Isolated dystonias: 1

## Young-onset generalized dystonia
- Onset is usually in late childhood/early teens.
- Also known as primary torsion dystonia or Oppenheim's dystonia.
- Limb (usually leg) onset of dystonia is typical, with spread of symptoms over months to 2 years, often resulting in generalized dystonia. However, some patients may only develop focal/segmental symptoms. Symptoms then typically plateau, and, although they may wax and wane, development of new dystonic symptoms should prompt re-evaluation of the diagnosis.
- Involvement of cranial and bulbar structures by dystonia is very unusual.
- Fifty to 60% of patients will have a mutation in the *TOR1A* gene on chromosome 9q.

## DYT1 dystonia

### Genetics
DYT1 dystonia is due to a GAG deletion in the *TOR1A* (torsin 1A) gene. The *TOR1A* gene codes for torsin A, a protein that probably has a chaperone function within the cell and is highly expressed within dopaminergic areas of the brain. The *TOR1A* deletion occurs in all ethnic groups but has a high prevalence in the Ashkenazi Jewish population because of a founder effect. Testing for the DYT1 mutation is technically easy and widely commercially available (see Video 9.1: DYT1 dystonia).

### Inheritance
DYT1 dystonia is inherited in an autosomal dominant fashion but has reduced penetrance; only 30% of mutation carriers develop symptoms. The penetrance is age-dependent; if a mutation carrier reaches the age of 25 without developing symptoms, they are unlikely ever to develop dystonia.

### Phenotype
The phenotype is as described on p. 204. While some patients develop severe generalized dystonia, others may just have mild focal dystonia of the limbs. Once the condition has plateaued, further progression is highly unusual. Long-term consequences of dystonic postures (scoliosis, nerve entrapment, spinal cord compression due to spondylosis) may occur.

### Non-DYT1 young-onset generalized dystonia
Some patients with young-onset generalized dystonia will be negative for the *TOR1A* mutation. Another cause of isolated generalized dystonia may be DYT6 (*THAP1* mutations) but typically has a different age and site of onset to DYT1 (see DYT6 dystonia, p. 205). Moreover, it is important in such patients to explore through history and examination any possibility of acquired/neurodegenerative dystonia and look for the development of new signs and symptoms at follow-up. In those patients who truly have isolated dystonia, the clinical phenotype and response to treatment is similar to patients with *TOR1A* mutations.

## DYT6 dystonia

### Genetics
DYT6 dystonia is due to *THAP1* gene mutations. *THAP1* shows significant mutational heterogeneity with currently over 60 different missense and truncating mutations, and no phenotype–genotype correlations have been found.

### Inheritance
DYT6 is inherited in an autosomal dominant manner, with penetrance estimated at 40%.

### Phenotype
The gene was first identified in three Mennonite families, who are related by a common ancestor dating to the mid 1700s who had adult-onset cranio-cervical dystonia. Since then, it has been identified worldwide. Usually the age of onset is later than in DYT1 dystonia (mean 19 years; range 5–38 years). Site of onset is either an upper limb or the cervical region, followed by laryngeal dystonia, and, in some, generalization may occur.

## Differential diagnosis
DRD is the most important differential diagnosis to consider, and a trial of levodopa is appropriate in all patients with young-onset dystonia. Some combined dystonias due to an inherited/sporadic neurodegenerative cause may have young onset and present initially with dystonia alone, e.g. WD (➔ p. 220), NBIA (➔ p. 224), and juvenile PD (➔ p. 42). Thus, when appropriate, a DAT scan may be needed to exclude juvenile PD.

## Investigations
In patients with young-onset (childhood, adolescence) isolated dystonia, the following investigations are appropriate if there are no pointers towards a possible secondary/degenerative cause:
- DYT1 gene testing
- Copper, ceruloplasmin, slit-lamp examination
- Brain MRI.

## Treatment
- Medical treatment is symptomatic and discussed in detail on ➔ p. 234.
- DBS of the GPi has replaced previous lesion operations. GPi stimulation appears to be very effective, with sustained benefit, and is discussed on ➔ p. 244.

## Isolated dystonias: 2

### Adult-onset isolated limb dystonia
- Age of onset is typically 25–35 years.
- Men are more often affected than women.
- Usually sporadic; rare families reported with *DYT1*, *DYT6*, or *GTPCH1* mutations, with onset in the teens and twenties.
- The commonest form is 'writer's cramp' where the patient describes abnormal postures affecting the hand while writing, but not while performing other tasks. The unaffected hand may show abnormal movements while the patient is writing—'mirror movements'. Many patients will develop dystonia associated with other tasks, a pattern that is sometimes referred to as 'complex writer's cramp'.
- Patients will often have a sensory trick; changing the size or texture of the pen barrel may improve symptoms temporarily (see Video 9.2: Writing dystonia).
- If patients learn to write with their other hand, about a third will also develop writer's cramp in that hand.
- Remission of symptoms is reported but is very rare.
- In contrast with writer's cramp where excessive writing is rarely a precipitant, other adult-onset limb dystonias are usually precipitated by excessive practice of a particular movement. These 'task-specific' dystonias have been reported in the arms of musicians, typists, golfers, and even chapatti makers.
- Abnormal postures of the affected limb may only occur during a particular task (e.g. playing a musical instrument). Sensory tricks often occur, e.g. changing the size of the grip on the bow may temporarily improve dystonia in a violinist (see Video 9.3: Musician's dystonia).
- Dystonia is often not severe in these task-specific dystonias, but, because of the precision required for performance of the task (particularly the case for musicians), the effect on function can be devastating.
- Following a period of rest from the precipitating task, dystonia may be reduced when the task is performed again but will quickly return to the original level of severity.
- Adult-onset leg dystonia has occasionally been reported as part of the phenotypes of isolated dystonia but is very rare, and is almost always due to an acquired/degenerative cause.

# Isolated dystonias: 3

## Adult-onset isolated cranio-cervical dystonia

*Torticollis (cervical dystonia, spasmodic torticollis)*
- Typical age at onset is around 45 years. Women are more often affected than men (see Video 9.4: Cervical dystonia).
- Usually starts with gradual onset of discomfort in the neck, followed by involuntary pulling of the head in a particular direction because of contraction of certain neck and shoulder muscles. Tremor, which is jerky and worsened by trying to turn the head into a normal position, is very common and can be the predominant clinical feature. Occasionally, dystonic posture or tremor of the arms may occur.
- Patients often have a sensory trick where they can touch one side of their face and partially relieve the muscle spasm. Patients often resort to holding their hands to their face all the time.
- Symptoms usually progress over 6–12 months and then plateau. Symptoms are usually worsened by anxiety (e.g. being in a social situation).
- Remission of symptoms occurs in 5–10% of patients (usually those with younger onset) and may be sustained.

*GNAL dystonia*
Mutations in the *GNAL* (guanine nucleotide-binding protein (G-protein), alpha-activating activity polypeptide, olfactory-type) gene cause cervical or cranial dystonia, with onset often in the thirties, however, with a broad age range (7–53 years). It is estimated that *GNAL* mutations may account for around 1% of all cases of focal or segmental dystonia involving the cranio-cervical region.

*ANO3 and CIZ1*
Mutations in these two genes have also been described to cause adult-onset cranio-cervical dystonia that can become segmental. With *ANO3* (anoctamin 3) mutations, tremor is quite a prominent feature. However, these genes have not been confirmed in further patients, apart from the families initially described, and need further confirmation.

## Oromandibular dystonia

This is dystonia affecting the muscles of mastication, often with some additional involvement of the platysma. It has a similar age at onset to torticollis, and women are more often affected than men. Initially, the muscle spasm may be triggered by speaking or chewing but later will occur spontaneously as well. A combination of blepharospasm and oromandibular dystonia is known as Meige or Brueghel syndrome. Isolated oromandibular dystonia can look very similar to the abnormal movements caused by long-term use of DRBs; therefore, a careful drug history needs to be taken in these patients (see Video 9.5: Meige syndrome).

## Laryngeal dystonia

This is dystonia affecting the vocal cords. It has a similar age at onset and sex ratio to torticollis. The commoner form is adductor dystonia where the vocal cords tend to be held together. This produces a strangled coarse voice with frequent variations in pitch. Less commonly, in abductor dystonia, the vocal cords are held apart, resulting in a whispering breathy voice.

### TUBB4A

A missense mutation in the *TUBB4A* gene has been found to cause 'whispering dysphonia' in the same Australian kindred by two groups. The age at onset is in the second to third decade, and the phenotype is that of laryngeal dysphonia, cranio-cervical dystonia that may generalize, and a 'hobby horse' gait. Although these mutations have not been found in other populations, and thus seem to be a rare cause of isolated dystonia, mutations in the same gene have been found to cause hypomyelination with atrophy of the basal ganglia and cerebellum (H-ABC), which is a rare leukoencephalopathy characterized by variable onset (from infancy to childhood), developmental delay, dystonia, choreoathetosis, rigidity, opisthotonus and oculogyric crises, progressive spastic tetraplegia, ataxia, and more rarely seizures. MRI shows a combination of hypomyelination, cerebellar atrophy, and absence or disappearance of the putamen.

## Blepharospasm

This is dystonia affecting the muscles around the eyes. It tends to have a slightly later age at onset, compared with other cranio-cervical dystonias (mean age at onset approximately 63 years). Women are more commonly affected than men. Patients frequently report a gritty or uncomfortable feeling in the eyes before the onset of the spasm in the orbicularis oculi. As well as the spasm closing the eyes, there is typically an inability to activate the levator palpebrae, so that the eyelid can open. This 'levator inhibition' is also seen in PSP.

## Investigation of isolated adult-onset dystonia

In a typical clinical scenario with no suggestion on history or examination of a secondary/degenerative cause, no investigation is needed. It is worthwhile considering:
- copper studies and slit-lamp examination in patients with onset under 50 years
- brain MRI
- cervical spine MRI if fixed or very painful dystonia (particularly laterocollis). MRI can miss atlanto-axial fractures/instability, and so a fine-cut CT through the upper cervical spine may also be necessary
- EMG of paraspinal muscles and anti-glutamic acid decarboxylase (GAD) antibodies if there is prominent axial spasm to exclude stiff person syndrome.

## Treatment

The mainstay of treatment for cranio-cervical dystonia is botulinum toxin, covered in detail on → p. 238. Treatment of writer's cramp and task-specific dystonia is difficult and is discussed on → p. 234.

## Combined dystonias: 1

Here, we will cover the combined dystonias that used to be called 'dystonia-plus syndromes'—DRDs and myoclonus dystonia. Myoclonus dystonia is discussed in detail on → p. 182.

### Dopa-responsive dystonia

DRD (DYT5a, Segawa syndrome) is a rare autosomal dominant condition which is entirely treatable with small doses of levodopa. If left untreated, severe disability can result.

#### Genetics

DRD is caused by mutations in the guanosine triphosphate cyclohydrolase 1 gene on chromosome 14q (*GTPCH1*). This enzyme is the rate-limiting step in the production of tetrahydrobiopterin (BH4), which is itself an essential cofactor for the production of dopamine from tyramine. If both *GTPCH1* genes are similarly homozygously mutated, patients usually present within 6 months with hyperphenylalaninaemia and severe neurological dysfunction. Infantile onset resembling cerebral palsy is uncommon and usually is due to compound heterozygous mutations. The metabolic pathway is shown in Fig. 9.1.

#### Phenotype

Typical age at onset is 2–5 years, with progressive limb dystonia, often with additional parkinsonism and spasticity. A common feature is diurnal variation, with symptoms becoming much worse as the day progresses. Girls are more commonly affected than boys (4:1).

DRD has a very variable presentation. Some patients have non-progressive arm dystonia, presenting in their twenties and mimicking simple writer's cramp. Most have severe symptoms with young onset, with additional apparent upper motor neuron signs on examination (brisk reflexes, spasticity, extensor plantar responses), mimicking cerebral palsy or hereditary spastic paraplegia. Because of the variability of presentation and the difficulty of diagnostic investigation, we recommend that all patients with young-onset dystonia (<25 years) receive a trial of levodopa.

#### Investigation

Genetic testing for mutations in the *GTPCH1* gene is not widely available. The gene is very large, and numerous mutations have been described, making genetic testing very difficult. Two alternative methods of diagnosis are currently used.

- **Phenylalanine loading test**: BH4 is required for the conversion of phenylalanine to tyramine, and therefore *GTPCH1* mutations cause impaired metabolism of phenylalanine. In the phenylalanine loading test, an oral dose of 100 mg/kg of phenylalanine is given, and phenylalanine levels are measured 1, 2, 4, and 6 hours post-dose. High post-dose phenylalanine levels are characteristic of DRD.
- **CSF pterin analysis**: it is possible to measure the levels of pterins (e.g. BH4 and neopterin-BH2) and dopamine and serotonin metabolites (5-hydroxyindoleacetic acid (5-HIAA) and homovanillic acid (HVA)) in the CSF. This test requires samples to be frozen

immediately after they are taken, and analysis is only available in a few specialist centres. In DRD, BH4, HVA, and 5-HIAA are all low. This type of CSF analysis has the advantage of screening for enzyme defects, other than *GTPCH1*, which may cause similar symptoms (Tables 9.4 and 9.5).

*Differential diagnosis*

Young-onset PD can present with dystonia and parkinsonism, which responds to levodopa, and therefore can cause some confusion with DRD. One would not wish to treat such patients with levodopa initially, and therefore differentiation is important. A dopamine transporter SPECT scan (DAT scan) is helpful here; it is normal in DRD, but abnormal in young-onset PD. However, in some adult-onset cases of parkinsonism and DRD mutations, the DAT scan may be abnormal, suggesting that *GTPCH1* may be a risk factor for the development of degenerative parkinsonism later on in life.

*Treatment*

Treatment is with levodopa. Typically, an excellent sustained response is achieved at small doses (200–400 mg of levodopa daily). Levodopa should be introduced slowly, as described in Chapter 3 (➔ p. 52). Long-term side effects of levodopa treatment which occur in PD (dyskinesia, on–off fluctuations) do not typically occur in DRD.

## Other childhood monoamine neurotransmitter disorders

There are a number of other monoamine neurotransmitter disorders that may occur mainly in childhood. These other conditions are recessive and cause younger-onset severe disease which may not respond fully to treatment. Tyrosine hydroxylase deficiency is a recessive condition causing parkinsonism, ptosis, myoclonic jerks, seizures, severe head lag, and truncal hypotonia. Levodopa is effective in treating these symptoms, but, if it is delayed, permanent disability may remain. CSF examination will reveal normal tetrahydrobiopterin and 5-HIAA levels, but almost unrecordable HVA levels. Patients with a similar presentation have also been reported with sepiapterin reductase deficiency (SRD). It can be helpful to think of the pterin pathway (Fig. 9.1) and the later stages of the monoamine synthesis pathway separately in order to help remember the different disorders. Table 9.4 shows these conditions and their phenotypes, and Table 9.5 shows the typical findings in the CSF that help to suspect these disorders.

## Dopamine transporter deficiency syndrome

Dopamine transporter deficiency is an autosomal recessive condition due to mutations of *SLC6A3* gene that encodes the dopamine transporter.
- Loss-of-function mutations lead to defective pre-synaptic uptake of dopamine, with accumulation of synaptic dopamine, which is then catabolized and results in the characteristic raised HVA levels in the CSF (Table 9.5).
- Clinically, age at onset is usually in infancy with irritability and axial hypotonia, adding later a progressive dystonic and dyskinetic movement disorder with eye involvement. During childhood, there is evolution of prominent parkinsonism, with death, in some patients, in adolescence.

## CHAPTER 9 **Dystonia**

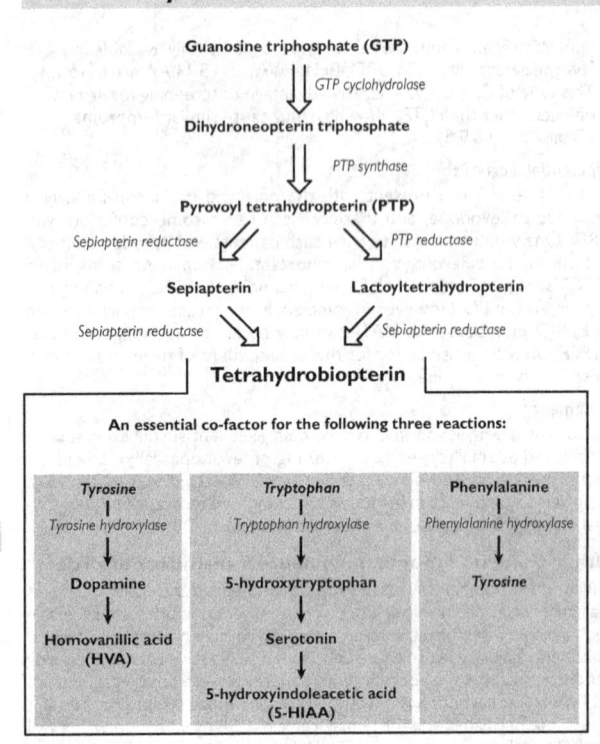

**Fig. 9.1** The pterin pathway.

- Adults with this syndrome are now recognized, presenting with parkinsonism; thus the disorder should be considered in the differential diagnosis of juvenile parkinsonism.
- The CSF neurotransmitter profile of raised CSF HVA:HIAA ratio of >5 is described in all reported cases, and this is the only disorder, to date, to have increased HVA.
- In contrast to DRD, the DAT scan is severely abnormal.
- The condition is unresponsive to currently available treatments, including levodopa, dopamine agonists, anticholinergics, benzodiazepines, and DBS.

**Table 9.4** Most important monoamine neurotransmitter disorders and their main clinical features

| | |
|---|---|
| GTPCH1 deficiency (AD, Segawa syndrome) | Dopa-responsive dystonia, classically with diurnal fluctuation, starting in the legs |
| GTPCH1 deficiency (AR) | Truncal hypotonia, dystonia, developmental delay, seizures |
| PTPS deficiency (pyruvoyl tetrahydropterin synthase) | Hypotonia, hypokinesia, rigidity, chorea, dystonia, oculogyric crisis |
| SRD deficiency (sepiapterin reductase) | Axial hypotonia, dystonia, oculogyric crisis, diurnal fluctuation |
| DHPR deficiency (dihydropteridine reductase) | Bulbar dysfunction, tremor, dystonia, choreoathetosis |
| TH deficiency (tyrosine hydroxylase) | Parkinsonism dystonia, focal or generalized dystonia, oculogyric crisis, tremor, ptosis, hypersalivation, autonomic disturbance |
| AADC deficiency | Hypotonia, oculogyric crisis, hypokinesia, chorea, dystonia, bulbar dysfunction |
| Dopamine transporter deficiency syndrome | Feeding difficulties, irritability, axial hypotonia, progressive dystonic and dyskinetic movement disorder with eye involvement |

**Table 9.5** Most important monoamine neurotransmitter disorders and the CSF findings in each of those

| Condition/ CSF | Phe | BH2 | BH4 | HVA | 5-HIAA | Others |
|---|---|---|---|---|---|---|
| GTP1 (AD) | N | ↓ | ↓ | ↓ | ↓/N | |
| GTP1 (AR) | ↑ | ↓ | ↓ | ↓ | ↓ | |
| PTPS | ↑ | N | ↓ | ↓ | ↓ | |
| SRD | N | ↑ | ↑ | ↓ | ↓ | |
| DHPR | ↑ | ↑ | ↑/N | ↓ | ↓ | ↓ folate |
| TH | N | N | N | ↓ | N | ↓ HVA/5HIAA ratio, ↑ serum prolactin |
| AADC | N | N | N | ↓ | ↓ | ↓ 3-methoxy-4-hydroxyphenylglycol |
| Dopamine transporter deficiency syndrome | N | N | N | ↑ | N | HVA:HIAA ratio >5 |

# Combined dystonias: 2

There are many degenerative neurological syndromes where dystonia occurs as just one of a number of symptoms and signs. A logical method with which to approach the investigation of patients with degenerative dystonia is to look for 'syndromic associations'—associated symptoms that help to narrow down the differential diagnosis. Table 9.6 lists the causes of degenerative dystonia with syndromic associations, and Table 9.7 gives diagnostic investigations for each condition. On the following pages, there is more detailed description of these conditions.

Table 9.6 Causes of combined dystonia due to degeneration

| | |
|---|---|
| Dystonia and parkinsonism | Parkinson's disease |
| | Progressive supranuclear palsy |
| | Multiple system atrophy |
| | Corticobasal degeneration |
| | Wilson's disease |
| | Huntington's disease |
| | Spinocerebellar ataxia (esp. SCA 3) |
| | GM1 gangliosidosis |
| | Neuronal brain iron accumulation syndrome |
| | Rapid-onset dystonia parkinsonism |
| | X-linked dystonia parkinsonism |
| | Dopa-responsive dystonias |
| | Dopamine transporter deficiency syndrome |
| Dystonia and eye movement disorder | Niemann–Pick type C |
| | Ataxia telangiectasia |
| | Ataxia oculomotor apraxia 1 and 2 |
| | Spinocerebellar ataxia |
| | Wilson's disease |
| | Huntington's disease |
| | Progressive supranuclear palsy |
| | Corticobasal degeneration |
| Dystonia with prominent bulbar involvement | Neuronal brain iron accumulation syndrome |
| | Neuroacanthocytosis |
| | Wilson's disease |

*(Continued)*

**Table 9.6** (Contd.)

| | |
|---|---|
| Dystonia with cerebellar ataxia | Spinocerebellar ataxia |
| | Ataxia telangiectasia |
| | AOA1, AOA2 |
| | Friedreich's ataxia |
| | Neuroacanthocytosis |
| | Wilson's disease |
| | Dentatorubropallidoluysian atrophy |
| | Multiple system atrophy |
| | Niemann–Pick type C |
| | Cervical dystonia and ataxia |
| | Huntington's disease |
| | GM2 gangliosidosis |
| Dystonia with peripheral neuropathy | Metachromatic leukodystrophy |
| | Spinocerebellar ataxia |
| | Neuroacanthocytosis |
| | GM2 gangliosidosis |
| Dystonia and deafness | Mohr–Tranebjaerg syndrome |
| | Woodhouse–Sakati syndrome |
| | Mitochondrial disorders |
| Other | Amino acidaemias (infantile-onset neurodevelopmental syndromes) |

**Table 9.7** Investigations that may be considered in the investigation of combined dystonia when a heredo-degenerative cause is suspected (testing should be guided by syndromic associations)

| | |
|---|---|
| Genetic tests | *Huntingtin* (Huntington's disease) |
| | *PANK2* gene (neuronal brain iron accumulation) |
| | *SCA1, 2, 3, 5, 7, 17* (spinocerebellar ataxia) |
| | Ferritin light chain (neuronal brain iron accumulation) |
| | *DRPLA* gene (dentatorubropallidoluysian atrophy) |
| | *NPC1/2* (Niemann–Pick type C) |
| | *ATM* (ataxia telangiectasia) |
| | *TIMM8A* (Mohr–Tranebjaerg syndrome) |
| | *ATP1A3* (rapid-onset dystonia parkinsonism) |
| | *TAF1* gene (X-linked dystonia parkinsonism) |
| Bloods | Acanthocytes (neuroacanthocytosis, neuronal brain iron accumulation) |
| | Copper, ceruloplasmin (Wilson's disease, neuronal brain iron accumulation) |
| | Plasma amino acids (amino acidaemias) |
| | White cell enzymes (GM1/2 gangliosidosis, metachromatic leukodystrophy) |
| | Alpha-fetoprotein (ataxia telangiectasia) |
| | Immunoglobulins (ataxia telangiectasia) |
| | CK (neuroacanthocytosis) |
| | Uric acid (Lesch–Nyhan) |
| Urine tests | Urinary organic acids (amino acidaemias) |
| | 24-hour urinary copper (Wilson's disease) |
| Brain MRI | Iron deposition (neuronal brain iron accumulation) |
| | Caudate atrophy (Huntington's disease) |
| | Leukodystrophy (metachromatic leukodystrophy) |
| | White matter—high signal (amino acidaemias) |
| Functional imaging | Abnormal DAT scan (Parkinson's disease, corticobasal degeneration, multiple system atrophy, progressive supranuclear palsy) |
| Other | Slit-lamp examination (Wilson's disease) |
| | Liver biopsy (Wilson's disease) |
| | Nerve conduction studies (metachromatic leukodystrophy, neuroacanthocytosis, spinocerebellar ataxia, GM2 gangliosidosis) |
| | Electroretinography (neuronal brain iron accumulation) |
| | Skin biopsy (filipin testing for Niemann–Pick type C) |

# Combined dystonias: 3

### Dystonia with parkinsonism
- **PD**: dystonia can occur as a presenting feature of PD (➔ p. 21), in young-onset PD (➔ p. 43), and as 'off' and 'on' period dystonia during treatment (➔ p. 78).
- **PSP**: axial dystonia and dystonia affecting levator palpebrae (levator inhibition) occurs in PSP (➔ p. 96).
- **MSA**: patients with MSA may develop dystonia affecting the neck, causing forward flexion (anterocollis), and laryngeal dystonia causing dysphonia and stridor. If given levodopa, MSA patients may develop dystonia of facial muscles (➔ p. 102).
- **CBD**: patients with CBD often present with, or develop, dystonia affecting one hand or foot. Some patients develop very severe, relatively fixed dystonia affecting the hand—a 'dystonic clenched fist' (➔ p. 108).
- **Rapid-onset dystonia parkinsonism**: a rare autosomal dominant condition caused by mutations in *ATP1A3* (*DYT12*)—a sodium/potassium channel gene. Rapid development of dystonia and parkinsonism occurs in young adults, often precipitated by infection or physical stress. Symptoms usually plateau after a month, but recovery is rare. Notably, mutations in this gene are responsible for up to 75% of cases with alternating hemiplegia of childhood (AHC).
- **X-linked dystonia parkinsonism (Lubag)**: an X-linked recessive condition due to mutations in *TAF1* gene, occurring mainly on the island of Panay in the Philippines. There is a variable age at onset (<50 years) of progressive generalized dystonia and parkinsonism. Levodopa responsiveness is seen in some patients.
- **GM1 gangliosidosis**: recessively inherited lysosomal storage disorder, usually of childhood onset, but adult onset occurs. In adult disease, there is progressive parkinsonism, dementia, and dystonia. White cell enzyme analysis shows low levels of beta-galactosidase.
- **DRDs** (➔ p. 210), in particular dopamine transporter deficiency syndrome.
- **NBIAs** (➔ p. 224), **WD** (➔ p. 220), **HD** (➔ p. 164), and **SCAs** (➔ p. 282) can all cause dystonia and parkinsonism.

### Dystonia with an eye movement disorder
- **Niemann–Pick type C**: an autosomal recessive disorder characterized by onset in childhood of a vertical supranuclear gaze palsy, ataxia, dystonia, and cognitive decline. Onset has been reported in adulthood where disease progression is much slower. The disorder is due to failure of lipid esterification because of mutations in the *NPC1* or *NPC2* genes.
- **AT**: an autosomal recessive disorder of DNA repair caused by mutations on *ATM* gene. Presentation is in childhood with progressive ataxia, dystonia and/or chorea, difficulty in initiating saccades and sustaining gaze, and susceptibility to infection and cancer. Alpha-fetoprotein levels are often high; immunoglobulins are often low. Diagnosis is by tests of DNA fragility and genetic testing.
- **WD** (➔ p. 220), **SCAs** (➔ p. 282), **HD** (➔ p. 164), and **PSP** (➔ p. 96) can all cause dystonia and an eye movement disorder.

## Dystonia with prominent bulbar involvement
- **NBIAs**, which include panthonate kinase-associated neurodegeneration (PKAN) and neuroferritinopathy, are important causes of dystonia with bulbar involvement and are discussed separately on ➲ p. 224.
- **Neuroacanthocytosis** (➲ p. 170) can cause prominent bulbar dystonia.

## Dystonia with ataxia
- **SCAs**: a number of SCAs cause dystonia as well as ataxia (➲ p. 282). **Progressive cervical dystonia and ataxia** is reported, not caused by known *SCA* mutations.
- **GM2 gangliosidosis**: recessively inherited lysosomal storage disorder, also known as Tay–Sachs and Sandhoff disease. Childhood onset common, but adult onset also occurs. Adult-onset disease causes progressive dystonia, dementia, ataxia, chorea, and motor neuropathy. White cell enzyme analysis shows low levels of hexosaminidase A.
- **WD** (➲ p. 220), **HD** (➲ p. 164), **MSA** (➲ p. 102), **DRPLA** (➲ p. 187), **neuroacanthocytosis** (➲ p. 170), **NBIA** (➲ p. 224), Niemann–Pick type C, AT, AOA1, and AOA2 can all cause dystonia and ataxia.

## Dystonia with peripheral neuropathy
- **Metachromatic leukodystrophy**: a lysosomal storage disorder characterized by progressive dystonia, ataxia, cognitive decline, and peripheral neuropathy. Onset is usually in childhood, but adult onset is well recognized. White cell enzyme analysis shows low levels of aryl sulfatase A, and white matter changes are seen on MRI.
- **SCAs** (➲ p. 282), **GM2 gangliosidosis** and **neuroacanthocytosis** (➲ p. 170) can cause neuropathy and dystonia.

## Dystonia and deafness
- **Mohr–Tranebjaerg syndrome** (X-linked dystonia–deafness): a syndrome of childhood-onset deafness, and later onset of progressive dystonia, spasticity, visual failure, and cognitive decline. The condition is X-linked recessive and is due to mutations of the *TIMM8A* gene.
- **Woodhouse–Sakati syndrome**: a rare autosomal recessive neuroendocrine disorder, characterized by alopecia, hypogonadism, diabetes mellitus, mental retardation, sensory neural deafness, dystonia, and chorea of the limbs, with onset in adolescence. Pyramidal signs and neuropathy. The condition is autosomal recessive and is caused by mutation of the *C2orf37* gene. In some acidaemias (e.g. methylmalonic aciduria) or mitochondrial conditions, the combination of dystonia and deafness may be seen.

## Others
- **Amino acidaemias**: various disorders of amino acid metabolism can cause dystonia as part of a much wider neurological dysfunction and developmental regression. Diagnosis is via urinary organic acid and plasma amino acid measurements. Acidaemias that can cause dystonia include glutaric acidaemia type 1 and methylmalonic acidaemia.

# Wilson's disease

It is difficult to choose the appropriate section in which to place the discussion of WD. It has a wide range of clinical presentations and often presents as a true 'mixed movement disorder'. Although it is a rare disorder, it is treatable and is fatal if left untreated.

Samuel Alexander Kinnear Wilson (1878–1937) studied medicine in Edinburgh and later worked at National Hospital for Neurology in London. In 1911, he published his doctoral thesis *Progressive lenticular degeneration: a familial nervous disease associated with cirrhosis of the liver*, followed a year later by a paper on the same subject in the journal *Brain*. He was a renowned teacher, introduced the word 'extrapyramidal' into the medical lexicon, and apparently preferred to call the disease he described 'Kinnear Wilson's disease'. He single-handedly wrote one of the finest textbooks of neurology. He died aged 59 from cancer.

## Epidemiology

WD is rare, with a prevalence of 30 per million. Higher rates are seen in South America, and males are more often affected than females. Age at onset is usually in late childhood/teens, but onset has been reported between ages 3 and 52 years and, rarely, even later.

## Pathophysiology

WD is an autosomal recessive condition due to a mutation in the copper transporting gene *ATP7B* on chromosome 13q. Numerous mutations have been described, which cause loss of function of the transporter protein and accumulation of toxic free copper within the body.

## Clinical features

There are two common presentations of WD.
- Hepatic presentation: young age at onset (mean: 11 years). Presents primarily with acute hepatic failure or signs of chronic liver disease.
- Neurological presentation: older age at onset (mean: 18 years). Presents primarily with neurological symptoms:
  - tremor: often a dramatic 'wing-beating' tremor present at rest, worse on posture, and much worse on action
  - dystonia
  - parkinsonism
  - cerebellar signs
  - gait disturbance: often gait is bizarre, caused by a combination of ataxia, dystonia, and chorea
  - psychiatric disturbance: may be the presenting feature of the condition and includes personality change, disinhibition, emotional lability, and progressive cognitive decline.
- Kayser–Fleischer rings: red–brown pigmentation around the edge of the iris due to deposition of copper in the Descemet's membrane. Best seen on slit-lamp examination.
- Sunflower cataract: radiating red–brown pattern of copper deposition in the lens.

Other features of WD include osteoporosis, haemolytic anaemia, pigment gallstones, renal stones, and skin hyperpigmentation.

## Diagnosis of Wilson's disease

Diagnosis of WD is complex, and, in cases where diagnostic suspicion is high, a liver biopsy may be the only method by which to conclusively prove or disprove the diagnosis. Gene analysis is usually impractical as a diagnostic tool, as so many mutations have been found, and many patients are 'compound heterozygotes', i.e. carry a different mutation on each WD gene. However, in certain populations, particular mutations are common and can be tested for. MRI of the brain may show generalized atrophy with a high T2 signal in the basal ganglia, but this is not specific for WD. Kayser–Fleischer rings are not always present and can occur in other chronic liver diseases. However, it is very rare for Kayser–Fleischer rings not to be found in patients with neurological WD on slit-lamp examination by an experienced ophthalmologist.

*Tests available for Wilson's disease*
- **Blood for copper and ceruloplasmin**: ceruloplasmin is a copper-transporting protein not coded for by the *WD* gene. Its level is usually low in WD, as copper is needed for its synthesis. This test estimates copper bound to ceruloplasmin, and therefore it is also low. However, levels of both can be normal in WD. Ceruloplasmin levels can be low in WD heterozygotes (1:900 people).
- **24-hour urinary copper**: this is more reliable than blood screening. It is typically >100 micrograms/24 hour in WD, but levels of >40 micrograms/24 hour are suggestive and indicate the need for further investigation.
- **Penicillamine challenge**: probably more reliable than simple 24-hour urinary copper estimation, but not proven for adult patients, and penicillamine can have acute side effects.
- **Liver biopsy**: this is the best method for conclusively diagnosing WD but is an invasive test with associated morbidity and mortality. Copper-free instruments and containers must be used. Liver copper content >250 micrograms/g dry weight of liver is considered diagnostic. In untreated patients, a level <40–50 micrograms/g excludes WD.

### How to do a penicillamine challenge
- Take 500 mg of penicillamine, and begin urine collection into copper-free containers.
- Twelve hours later, take further 500 mg of penicillamine.
- Finish the 24-hour urine collection.
- A penicillamine challenge will increase the urinary copper excretion in normal people; therefore, normal ranges for 24-hour urinary copper excretion do not apply. For a penicillamine challenge, a urinary copper excretion of >1600 micrograms/24 hours suggests WD.

# Treatment of Wilson's disease

- Two copper-chelating drugs (penicillamine and trientine) have been shown to be effective in WD. Tetrathiomolybdate is a newer chelating agent which may also be effective (may not be readily available in the UK).
- Zinc may also be used. It can be used as first-line therapy but is more often given after the disease has been stabilized with copper-chelating drugs. Copper chelators also chelate zinc; therefore, combined prescription may well reduce the effectiveness of zinc and vice versa. Zinc encourages the formation of proteins in the intestinal mucosa which bind both zinc and copper, holding them within the mucosa until it is sloughed off.
- Patients with fulminant hepatic failure or severe chronic liver disease may require transplantation.
- Monitoring of treatment efficacy and compliance is essential and is usually achieved by periodic 24-hour urinary copper measurement.

## Strategy

- Copper-chelating agents are essential but may have significant side effects—this is particularly the case for penicillamine.
- Trientine has fewer side effects than penicillamine and therefore is a rational first-line therapy. Tetrathiomolybdate is another alternative to penicillamine, although evidence regarding its use is limited. However, it does appear to have fewer side effects than penicillamine.
- Patients will usually be able to stop or reduce the dose of chelating agents after a period of initial treatment, and then start on zinc as maintenance therapy.
- Nuts, shellfish, chocolate, and mushrooms all contain high levels of copper and should be avoided.

### How to introduce medications commonly used for the treatment of Wilson's disease

*Trientine*

- Available in 300 mg tablets.
- Perform full blood count prior to treatment initiation.
- Initial dose 300 mg four times daily.
- Measure 24-hour urinary copper and full blood count weekly.
- Titrate dose according to urinary copper levels. Maximum dose 2.4 g daily.
- Main side effects include nausea, bone marrow suppression, and rash.

## Penicillamine

- Available in 125 mg and 250 mg tablets.
- Perform full blood count and urine dipstick prior to treatment.
- Starting dose is 500 mg tds.
- Measure 24-hour urinary copper, full blood count, and urine dipstick weekly during first 2 months of treatment.
- Titrate dose according to urinary copper levels. Maximum dose 2 g daily.
- Penicillamine should be given with pyridoxine 25 mg daily.
- Acute severe worsening of symptoms may occur with treatment initiation. Other important side effects include aplastic anaemia, immune complex nephritis, rash, nausea, and lupus-like syndrome.
- Patients who are allergic to penicillin may have anaphylaxis with penicillamine.

## Zinc

- Available in effervescent 125 mg tablets (containing 45 mg of zinc).
- Dose is one tablet tds.
- Main side effects are abdominal pain and dyspepsia.

# Neuronal brain iron accumulation syndromes

## From Hallervorden–Spatz to neuronal brain iron accumulation syndrome

In the 1920s, two German pathologists Julius Hallervorden and his boss Hugo Spatz described patients (mainly children) with progressive movement disorder associated with iron deposition within the basal ganglia. The term Hallervorden–Spatz syndrome was coined to describe this rather heterogenous group of patients. It has since come to light that Julius Hallervorden was involved in unethical experimentation during Nazi control of Germany, and therefore the name of the condition has been changed to neuronal brain iron accumulation syndrome (NBIA).

## Causes of neuronal brain iron accumulation syndrome

### Current classification of causes of neuronal brain iron accumulation syndrome

- Pantothenate kinase-associated neurodegeneration (PKAN, NBIA type I), *PANK2* gene mutations, AR.
- Phospholipase 2, group VI-associated neurodegeneration (PLAN, NBIA type II; INAD1), *PLA2G6* gene mutations, AR.
- Mitochondrial membrane protein-associated neurodegeneration (MPAN), *C19orf12* mutations, AR.
- Fatty acid hydroxylase-associated neurodegeneration (FAHN), *FAH2* mutations, AR.
- Beta-propeller protein-associated neurodegeneration (BPAN), *WDR45* mutations, X-linked.
- Kufor–Rakeb syndrome, *ATP13A2* mutations, AR.
- Woodhouse–Sakati syndrome.
- Aceruloplasminaemia.
- Neuroferritinopathy; hereditary ferritinopathy; NBIA type III.
- COASY protein-associated neurodegeneration (CoPAN).

*Pantothenate kinase-associated neurodegeneration (PKAN, NBIA type I)*
Mutations in the pantothenate kinase 2 gene (*PANK2*) are responsible for about 50% of cases of NBIA (see Video 9.6: PANK2). Pantothenate kinase is involved in coenzyme A synthesis. Two main phenotypes are recognized.
- 'Classic' PKAN: onset in first decade of life (mean age 3.5 years) of progressive generalized dystonia, often with bulbar involvement, spasticity, and retinal degeneration (two-thirds of patients). Recessive.
- 'Atypical' PKAN: onset in first three decades of life (mean 13 years). Much more variable presentation with gait disturbance (freezing of gait described, spasticity, dystonia), behavioural disturbance, progressive generalized dystonia, and tics. Retinal degeneration is rare. Recessive.

In both classic and atypical forms of PKAN, MRI will almost always show a typical pattern of abnormality called 'the eye of the tiger'. This is seen on a T2-weighted axial scan as a central region of T2 hyperintensity in the globus pallidus surrounded by an area of T2 hypointensity (Fig. 9.2). This pattern is hardly ever seen in patients with other causes of NBIA (where T2 hypointensity alone is seen in the globus pallidus). Therefore, the 'eye of the tiger' sign is almost pathognomonic for *PANK2* mutations.

*Phospholipase 2, group VI-associated neurodegeneration (PLAN, NBIA type II; INAD1; Karak syndrome)*

*PLA2G6* gene mutations cause PLAN (NBIA type II). The encoded protein is a group VIA calcium-independent phospholipase A2 involved in the generation of free fatty acids and lysophospholipids.

Similar to PKAN, an age-dependent phenotype has been recognized.

- Early-onset cases develop infantile neuroaxonal dystrophy (INAD), characterized by progressive motor and mental retardation, marked truncal hypotonia, cerebellar ataxia, pyramidal signs, and early visual disturbances due to optic atrophy.
- Later onset may present milder, e.g. with complicated dystonia parkinsonism, sensitive to levodopa.

Early-onset cases show profound cerebellar involvement on neuroimaging. Half of INAD patients initially lack signs of iron accumulation in early disease stages but usually develop these throughout, affecting the globus pallidus. The central hyperintensity seen in PKAN is missing. In late-onset cases, iron may be absent, and MRI may even be completely normal. Others may show cortical atrophy or white matter changes. Pathology shows widespread alpha-synuclein-positive Lewy bodies as well as hyperphosphorylated tau.

*Mitochondrial membrane protein-associated neurodegeneration (MPAN)*

Mutations in *C19orf12* were identified as a cause of NBIA in a Polish cohort.

- Childhood-onset dysarthria and gait difficulty, followed by spastic paraparesis, dystonia and parkinsonism, neuropathy, optic atrophy, and psychiatric symptoms. Some patients may show similarity to juvenile ALS. Also mild phenotypes resembling idiopathic PD have been reported.
- Neuroimaging demonstrates iron accumulation in the globus pallidus and notably substantia nigra.
- Lewy body-like inclusions and hyperphosphorylated tau is seen in pathology.

*FA2H-associated neurodegeneration (FAHN)/SPG35*

*FA2H* mutations cause leukodystrophy, a form of hereditary spastic paraplegia (HSP) and overlapping syndromes, including atypical adult-onset spastic paraplegia, but also an NBIA phenotype.

- Patients present with childhood-onset gait impairment, spastic quadriparesis, severe ataxia, and dystonia. Seizures and divergent strabismus may be present.
- Brain imaging shows bilateral globus pallidus T2 hypointensities, consistent with iron deposition, prominent pontocerebellar atrophy,

mild cortical atrophy, white matter lesions, and corpus callosum thinning. Radiological overlap with leukodystrophies (white matter changes) and spastic paraplegias (thin corpus callosum) may be helpful clues when interpreting the MRI.
- Like other NBIA syndromes, the metabolic pathway of FA2H involves lipid and ceramides where it is important for myelin metabolim.

### Beta-propeller protein-associated neurodegeneration (BPAN)

NBIA cases with a homogenous clinical phenotype and disease history (known as SENDA—static encephalopathy of childhood with neurodegeneration in adulthood) have been linked to mutations in the *WDR45* gene.
- The course of the disease occurs in two stages, with developmental delay and intellectual disability in childhood and a second phase of rapid neurological deterioration characterized by parkinsonism and dementia.
- MRI shows clear sign of iron accumulation involving the substantia nigra and globus pallidus. A common and distinctive feature on T1-weighted imaging is the presence of a thin line of hypointensity in the substantia nigra and cerebral peduncles, surrounded by a hyperintense halo. Cerebral, and sometimes cerebellar, atrophy is present.
- The pathology shows iron accumulation in the substantia nigra and, to a lesser extent, the globus pallidus, axonal spheroids, gliosis, and neuronal loss. In the cerebellum, there is a significant reduction of Purkinje cells. Neurofibrillary tangles are present in different brain regions, while no positivity for alpha-synuclein or APP deposition was evident.
- BPAN is due to 'de novo' mutations in the *WDR45* gene causing loss of function of the encoded protein; even though the gene is on the X chromosome, both males and females present the same clinical phenotype, which seems to be due to somatic mosaicism or skewing of the X chromosome inactivation.

### Kufor–Rakeb syndrome

Mutations in *ATP13A2* cause Kufor–Rakeb disease.
- Kufor–Rakeb is characterized by early-onset levodopa-responsive parkinsonism, pyramidal signs, supranuclear upgaze palsy, and dementia. Oculogyric dystonic spasms, facial-faucial-finger mini-myoclonus, and autonomic dysfunction may be present. Psychiatric features include visual hallucinations.
- Brain imaging shows generalized atrophy, in addition to putaminal and caudate iron deposition, but not in all cases.
- The protein is a lysosomal 5 P-type ATPase. The role of the lysosome is supported by functional studies, leading to alpha-synuclein accumulation.
- Brain pathology is not available from any patient diagnosed with Kufor–Rakeb disease. However, *ATP13A2* mutations have been identified in a family with juvenile NCL.

### Aceruloplasminaemia

This is an autosomal recessive disorder caused by mutations in the gene encoding ceruloplasmin. Patients typically present in the third and fourth decades with a triad of retinal degeneration, diabetes, and neurological symptoms, typically dystonia, ataxia, and parkinsonism. There is absent ceruloplasmin, high serum ferritin, and iron deposition in the basal ganglia, but not in the 'eye of the tiger' pattern. Genetic testing is not generally available. There are anecdotal reports of benefit from treatment with iron-chelating agents (e.g. desferrioxamine) and fresh frozen plasma.

### Neuroferritinopathy
This is an autosomal dominant disorder caused by mutations in the ferritin light chain gene. It has only been reported, to date, in families from the UK and northern France. The typical age at onset is in the thirties to forties with progressive generalized dystonia, parkinsonism, chorea, and spasticity. Late onset with cognitive decline has also been reported. Patients generally have low serum ferritin, and iron deposition within the basal ganglia (but not of the 'eye of the tiger' type).

### Neuronal brain iron accumulation syndrome unclassified
A number of patients with a movement disorder and iron deposition in the basal ganglia will not have the known causes for their disorder and are currently denoted as NBIA unclassified.

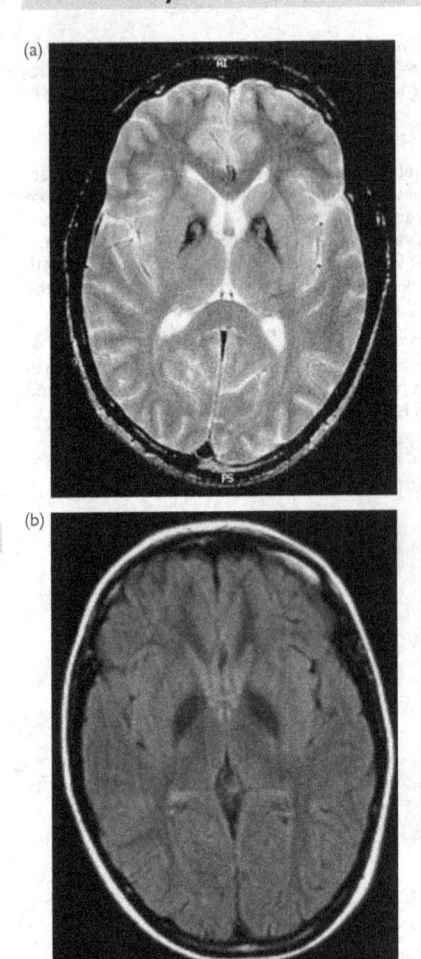

**Fig. 9.2** (a) The eye of the tiger sign in a patient with the *PANK2* mutation( note the bilateral globus pallidus hypointensity with a small area of hyperintensity within it on this T2-weighted MRI scan. (b) MRI of a patient with MPAN (note the bilateral globus pallidus hypointensity without the hyperintensity seen in *PANK2*) (we thank Dr Petr Dusek and Susanne Schneider for providing this figure).

# Acquired dystonia

These forms of dystonia (used to be called secondary) are due to environmental, iatrogenic, or traumatic causes. The key feature of these conditions is the presence of a precipitating event. It is important to remember that dystonia can sometimes develop some time after the original incident.

## Dystonia due to drugs

This topic is covered in detail in Chapter 10 (→ p. 254). In summary, a large number of prescribed drugs and drugs of abuse can cause *acute dystonic reactions* (ADRs)—dystonia usually affecting the face or neck, occurring shortly after drug exposure. DRBs can also cause *tardive dystonia*—dystonia that develops after chronic exposure to such drugs and often persists, even if the drug is stopped.

## Dystonia due to brain injury

Dystonia is associated with lesions of the basal ganglia, particularly the putamen. Hemidystonia often occurs with unilateral lesions. A common cause is vascular injury due to stroke. Hypoxic damage to the brain, particularly in the perinatal period, can cause severe generalized dystonia (often with spasticity). This presentation in children is often called 'athetoid cerebral palsy' and may develop some months after the original brain injury.

## Dystonia due to infection

Some patients with encephalitic illnesses can subsequently develop dystonia. Japanese B encephalitis, which can also cause post-infectious parkinsonism, is a well-recognized cause (→ p. 121). Encephalitis lethargica (→ p. 121) can also manifest as dystonia. Brain abscesses, if located in the basal ganglia, can produce dystonia in the same way as other structural lesions.

## Status dystonicus

Status dystonicus is a neurological emergency where a patient, typically with pre-existing dystonia, suffers from an acute and severe exacerbation of dystonia. There is often a precipitating factor such as a recent infection or drug changes. Dystonic spasms can be very severe and often cause bulbar and respiratory compromise.

### Treatment

Patients should be managed in a high-dependency or intensive care setting. Rhabdomyolysis and subsequent renal failure can occur as a result of prolonged muscle spasm. Treatment is difficult and is primarily supportive, together with benzodiazepines, anticholinergics, chemoparalysis, and ventilation. Some patients have been successfully treated acutely with pallidotomy and with DBS. However, most patients will recover spontaneously with adequate supportive treatment.

# Treatment of dystonia: strategies

Treatment of dystonia relies on four main methods:
- medical—drugs such as trihexyphenidyl and benzodiazepines
- botulinum toxin
- brain surgery—lesion operations and now DBS
- physical and 'retraining' therapies.

These treatments are not all suitable for every type of dystonia. Treatment strategies for different types of dystonia are given, and each method of treatment is considered in more detail on subsequent pages.

## Isolated young-onset generalized dystonia

- A trial of levodopa is appropriate in all patients with young-onset primary dystonia to exclude the possibility of DRD. Levodopa should be introduced in the way described in Chapter 3 (→ p. 52), and a dose of 300–600 mg/day taken for at least 2 months before effectiveness is judged.
- If, as is usually the case, levodopa is ineffective, the patient should start on trihexyphenidyl. Second-line treatments which may be of benefit include clonazepam, tetrabenazine, and baclofen. In severe disease, a combination of trihexyphenidyl, a DRB, and/or tetrabenazine, and sometimes clonazepam, can be helpful.
- Botulinum toxin has a limited role in patients with generalized dystonia. Isolated aspects of the dystonia, such as dystonia affecting the dominant hand, may be treated with botulinum toxin, with some functional benefit.
- DBS of the GPi can be of remarkable and sustained benefit to patients with isolated dystonia. It is rapidly emerging as a treatment to be considered early, particularly in patients with severe isolated generalized dystonia. It has replaced basal ganglia lesion operations such as pallidotomy and thalamotomy.

## Isolated adult-onset limb dystonia

- Consider a trial of levodopa in young-onset patients (<25 years), especially if there is a positive family history.
- Trihexyphenidyl is sometimes of benefit. Other medical treatments only rarely offer any benefit.
- Botulinum toxin may be of benefit but usually requires specialized administration under EMG guidance. It commonly causes excessive weakness of the hand, which limits the functional benefit of injections. This is particularly the case for those with task-specific dystonias where the task which precipitates the dystonia requires fine motor control (e.g. musicians).
- A number of 'motor retraining' strategies, such as constraint-induced movement therapy, have been trialled on a research basis, with some success reported.
- DBS of the GPi may be of benefit to these patients, but few cases have been reported.

### Isolated adult-onset cranio-cervical dystonia
- Botulinum toxin is the first-line treatment for patients with cervical dystonia or blepharospasm. Occasionally, such patients will respond to trihexyphenidyl. Patients with significant head tremor often respond to small doses of clonazepam.
- Oromandibular dystonia is best treated by botulinum toxin injections, but weakness around the mouth (causing swallowing difficulties and drooling) is a common side effect. Such injections require specialist EMG guidance.
- Laryngeal dystonia can be treated by EMG-guided injections in a specialist setting. Swallowing problems and hypophonia are common side effects.

### Combined dystonias due to a secondary cause
- Treatment of ADRs and tardive dystonia is discussed in Chapter 10 (➲ p. 256).
- Treatment of dystonia secondary to brain injury or post-encephalitis is similar to medical treatment of young-onset isolated dystonia. Botulinum toxin can be used to treat focal disabling areas of dystonia. Some patients with severe generalized dystonia due to brain injury (e.g. athetoid cerebral palsy) have received DBS of the GPi. Response is often very limited, compared with the results in isolated dystonia, but may still be of functional benefit.

### Combined dystonias due to heredo-degenerative disorders
- Dystonia is often only one of a number of symptoms in these conditions and may not require specific treatment.
- If treatment is needed, medical treatment as for young-onset isolated dystonia is given in combination with botulinum toxin injections for certain localized problems (e.g. hand dystonia). DBS of the GPi has a limited role in these patients, and response is much less than is seen in young-onset isolated dystonia.

# Treatment of dystonia: medical

The drugs listed in the box are sometimes of benefit in the treatment of dystonia. In severe dystonia, combinations of these drugs can be used. Slow titration of doses is essential to limit side effects.

### Trihexyphenidyl (benzhexol)
- Available as generic tablets: 2 mg and 5 mg (white, scored) or in syrup (5 mg/5 mL).
- Starting dose is 1 mg daily. Increase by 1 mg every 4–7 days to reach 1 mg tds. Then increase by 1 mg every 4–7 days to reach 2–4 mg tds.
- If side effects occur, dose titration should be stopped and then re-attempted after 1–2 weeks. Maximum dose may be as high as 50–100 mg daily.*
- Common side effects are dry mouth, dry eyes, nausea, confusion, constipation, and urinary retention.
- Important contraindication: closed-angle glaucoma.

### Clonazepam
- Available in 500 micrograms (beige) or 2 mg (white) tablets. Tablets scored twice.
- Starting dose is 250 micrograms once daily (125 micrograms in the elderly).
- Increase by 250 micrograms every week to reach 500 micrograms to 1 mg bd or tds.
- Maximum dose 4–6 mg daily.
- Main side effects are sedation, depression, and fatigue.

### Tetrabenazine
- Available in 25 mg tablets (yellow-buff, scored).
- Starting dose is 12.5 mg once daily.
- Increase every week by 12.5 mg to reach 12.5 mg tds, and then increase in 12.5 mg increments to reach 25–50 mg tds, as symptoms require.
- Maximum dose 200 mg daily.
- Main side effects are parkinsonism and depression.

### Baclofen
- Available in 10 mg tablets (scored) and as liquid (5 mg/5 mL).
- Starting dose is 5 mg at night.
- Increase dose by 5 mg every week to reach 10 mg tds.
- Maximum dose 100 mg daily.
- Main side effects are sedation, nausea, dizziness, and confusion.
- Baclofen should not be discontinued suddenly.

##  TREATMENT OF DYSTONIA: MEDICAL

# Treatment of dystonia: botulinum toxin 1

## Botulinum toxin

Botulinum toxin (BT) is produced by the anaerobic organism *Clostridium botulinum* and was previously a common cause of fatal food poisoning. It works by blocking neuromuscular transmission. In nature, there are seven subtypes of BT (A–G), each producing neuromuscular blockade by interfering with a different protein involved in pre-synaptic function. Commercially produced BT is either of subtype A or subtype B.

## Preparations and administration

Four types of BT are available commercially: Botox® (BT type A), Dysport® (BT type A), Xeomin® (BT type A), and Neurobloc® (BT type B) (known as Myobloc® in the United States) (Table 9.8).

- Commercially available BT has large differences in potency, and doses are NOT equivalent.
- Table 9.8 shows equivalent doses. However, these are a guide only, and considerable debate exists as to the correct conversion.
- Great care should be taken when switching toxin, as individual differences between patients may greatly affect the potency of different toxins. BT is given by intramuscular injection, using a 22- or 24-gauge needle, into muscles affected by dystonic spasm.
- BT works by weakening the muscle, thereby reducing the muscle spasm.
- Localization of the muscle is usually by using anatomical landmarks, but, in some cases (e.g. injection of forearm muscles for hand dystonia), EMG guidance of injection is used.
- BT usually takes 2–3 days to start working, has its peak effect by 2 weeks, and wears off in approximately 2–4 months. Therefore, repeat injections are necessary to maintain effect.

Table 9.8 Types of botulinum toxin

|  | Botox® | Dysport® | Xeomin® | Neurobloc®/Myobloc® |
|---|---|---|---|---|
| BT serotype | A | A | A | B |
| Mechanism of action | Cleaves SNAP25 | Cleaves SNAP25 | Cleaves SNAP25 | Cleaves VAMP |
| Provided as | Vial containing 100 MU in powder form | Vial containing 500 MU or 300 MU in powder form | Vial containing 100 MU in powder form | Vial containing 2500, 5000, or 10 000 MU in liquid form |
| Reconstitution | With normal saline | With normal saline | With normal saline | Available reconstituted |
| Storage | 2–8°C | 2–8°C | Room temperature | Room temperature |
| Equivalent dose | 1 MU* | 3–4 MU* | 1 MU* | 50 MU* |

SNAP25, synaptosomal associated protein 25; VAMP, vesicle-associated membrane protein (also called synaptobrevin 2).

## Side effects
- Excessive weakness of muscles injected, e.g. injection of posterior neck muscles causing head drop, injection of orbicularis oculi causing ptosis.
- Spread of effect to adjacent muscles. Particularly important in anterior neck injections (e.g. sternomastoid), with spread to pharyngeal muscles causing swallowing problems.
- Local bruising and pain due to injection.
- Allergic reactions (very rare).
- Autonomic side effects (dry mouth, dry eyes, urinary symptoms) occur with BT type B and, to a lesser extent, BT type A.
- Systemic botulism has not been reported with current toxins. The dose needed to cause systemic botulism is 20–30 times the maximum dose used clinically.

## Resistance
A small percentage of patients chronically treated with BT will develop circulating antibodies to the toxin, rendering it ineffective. Factors which appear to increase the rates of resistance include the following:
- longer duration of treatment
- higher doses of BT (e.g. resistance has never been reported with treatment for blepharospasm where doses used are approximately 10% of those used for cervical dystonia)
- higher frequency of injection.

### Diagnosis of resistance
- In the laboratory, by injection into mice of a lethal dose of BT mixed with serum from the patient.
- A dose of BT injected into the patient's extensor digitorum brevis, with EMG assessment of maximum muscle contraction before and 2 weeks after injection. Less than 50% reduction in EMG amplitude 2 weeks following injection suggests resistance to BT.

### Managing resistance—a difficult problem
- Patients resistant to BT type A may respond to BT type B. However, many patients have antibodies which cross-react with types A and B. Independent resistance to BT type B can also occur.
- Antibody titres slowly reduce over time when BT exposure is stopped, but may take years.
- Anecdotal reports of immunosuppression and plasma exchange for management of resistance exist, but effectiveness is limited.

### Avoiding resistance
- Use the smallest dose of toxin necessary to achieve effect.
- Maximum frequency of injections every 10–12 weeks.
- Avoid 'booster' injections.

### Botulinum toxin has stopped working—why?
- Incorrect injection placement.
- Wrong muscles injected.
- Dose error.
- Insufficient dose.
- Resistance.

# Treatment of dystonia: botulinum toxin 2

## Cervical dystonia

Head position in cervical dystonia depends on the pattern of muscle spasm. Table 9.9 gives a list of the common head positions in cervical dystonia and the muscles that are usually involved and which therefore may be injected with BT. Clinically, one can also classify according to the muscles involved in -caput or -collis (atlanto-occipital joints; latero- or torti-caput), or only muscles which work on the cervical spine (latero- or torti-collis). Fig. 9.3 shows the anatomy of these muscles.

Table 9.9 Common head positions and muscles responsible in cervical dystonia

| Dystonia pattern | Description | Muscles usually involved |
|---|---|---|
| Anterocollis | Head flexed forwards | Bilateral sternomastoid (bilateral sternomastoid injections can cause severe dysphagia), scalenes |
| Torticollis | Head turning | Ipsilateral splenius capitis, trapezius, contralateral sternomastoid |
| Laterocollis | Head tilted to the side | Ipsilateral sternomastoid, splenius capitis, and scalenes |
| Retrocollis | Head tipped backwards | Bilateral semispinalis, splenius capitis |

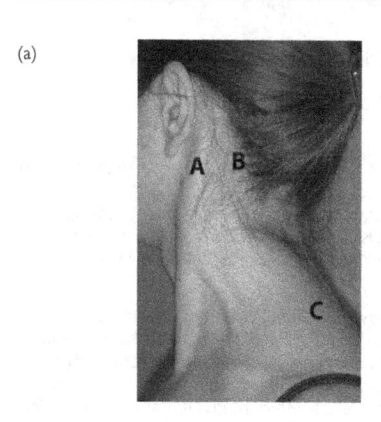

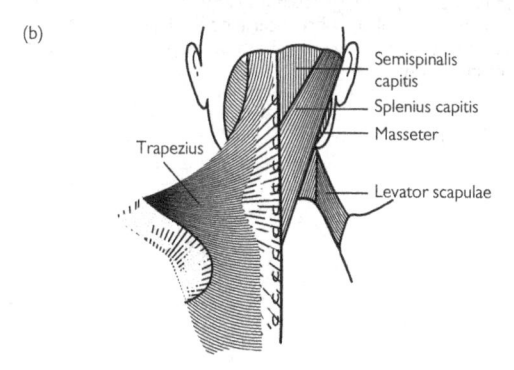

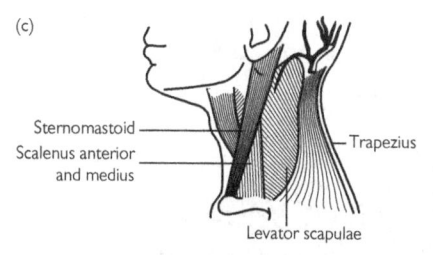

**Fig. 9.3** Muscle anatomy of the neck and approximate botulinum toxin injection sites. (a) Photograph of the neck from the side, with the head turned to the right: A, site commonly used for sternomastoid injection; B, site commonly used for splenius capitis injection; C, site commonly used for trapezius injection. Note that the right splenius capitis is best felt with the patient's head turned towards the right. (b), (c) Anatomical drawings of the neck muscles from the back and the side.

# Treatment of dystonia: botulinum toxin 3

### Blepharospasm
Fig. 9.4 shows the anatomy of the muscles around the eye, with common injection sites marked.

For the majority of patients, an injection above and lateral to, and below and lateral to, the eye is sufficient. Injections medial and inferior to the eye may spread to affect the lacrimal gland, causing dry eyes.

#### Levator inhibition
Some patients have blepharospasm due to dystonia affecting the pretarsal portion of the orbicularis oculi (Fig. 9.4). Such patients have very little spasm around the eyes; instead their eyelids simply close and often have to be opened by hand. This pattern of blepharospasm is more usually seen in the setting of PSP and, less commonly, PD. It is sometimes called 'apraxia of eyelid opening', although it is not clear that it fulfils the criteria for an apraxia, and is most likely subcortical in origin. Injections into the pretarsal portion of the orbicularis oculi can be helpful (see Video 9.7: PSP levator inhibition).

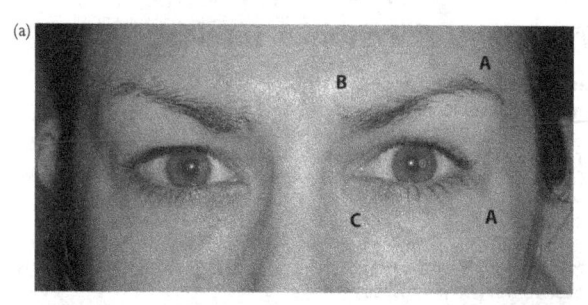

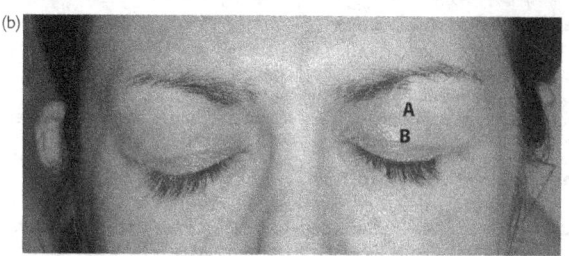

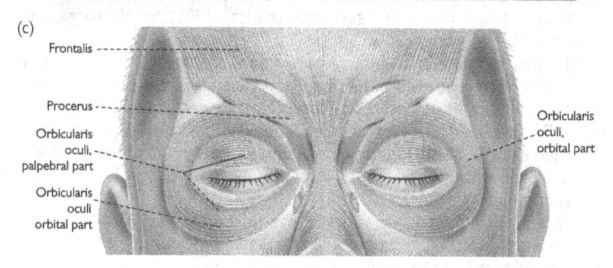

**Fig. 9.4** (a) Patient with eyes open: A, the two sites most commonly injected for blepharospasm; B, C, additional sites that are occasionally used. (b) Patient with eyes closed: A, site for preseptal injections; B, site for pretarsal injections. (c) Anatomical drawing of the muscles around the eye.

# Treatment of dystonia: surgical

## Peripheral operations
A number of peripheral procedures have been used in the past in an attempt to treat cervical dystonia and blepharospasm. These procedures generally had limited success and now are rarely used.
- Cervical rhizotomy: section of cervical roots supplying dystonic neck muscles.
- Selective peripheral denervation: section of nerve branches to dystonic muscles in the neck or face.
- Muscle stripping: resection of some muscle fibres from the orbicularis oculi to treat blepharospasm.

## Central lesion operations
Pallidotomy and, more rarely, thalamotomy have been used as treatment for dystonia. Bilateral pallidotomy can be beneficial in treatment of severe generalized dystonia, but risks from the operation (e.g. dysarthria, dysphagia) are notable. These lesion operations have largely been replaced by DBS.

## Deep brain stimulation
In this procedure, electrodes are inserted into the GPi under stereotactic guidance. The wires are then tunnelled underneath the skin and attached to a subcutaneously implanted stimulator.

This procedure has been used since the late 1990s for dystonia, and results in isolated young-onset generalized dystonia have been extremely good, with sustained 70–80% improvement in symptoms commonly reported. Recent studies have suggested that DBS may also be effective for isolated adult-onset focal dystonias, in particular cervical dystonia. Results have been less impressive in dystonia due to brain injury or degenerative disease. Stimulators are expensive, and they require specialized surgical techniques to insert them and specialist follow-up to adjust stimulator settings.

Side effects include brain injury at the time of operation, lead infection, and lead fracture. Replacement of the stimulator battery is required every few years (via a local anaesthetic procedure).

# TREATMENT OF DYSTONIA: SURGICAL

# Treatment of dystonia: physical and 'retraining' therapies

Patients with task-specific dystonias may respond to methods of movement 'retraining'. Such therapies are largely available on a research basis only. The main focus of such therapies is to try to restore independent movement of each of the fingers. This is achieved in some techniques by restraining other fingers, while one finger is moved by the patient (constraint-induced movement therapy). Other techniques try to retrain the sensory system by teaching tasks that require a high degree of sensory discrimination (e.g. learning Braille). At present, the value of these and other retraining therapies remains uncertain, and further data are awaited.

# Useful websites and addresses

- **The Dystonia Society (UK)**: 2nd Floor, 89 Albert Embankment, London, SE1 7TP. Tel: 020 7793 3658; Helpline: 020 7793 3651; http://www.dystonia.org.uk.
- **Dystonia Medical Research Foundation (DMRF)-USA**: http://www.dystonia-foundation.org.
- **The Bachmann–Strauss Dystonia & Parkinson Foundation (USA)**: http://www.dystonia-parkinsons.org.
- **Benign Essential Blepharospasm Research Foundation (USA)**: http://www.blepharospasm.org/.
- **National Spasmodic Torticollis Association (USA)**: http://www.torticollis.org.
- **Dopa-Responsive Dystonia Central (USA)**: http://www.drdcentral.com.
- **Wilson's Disease Support Group UK**: http://www.wilsonsdisease.org.uk/WDSG-P0.asp.
- **Wilson Disease Association (USA)**: http://www.wilsonsdisease.org.
- **NBIA Disorders Association (USA)**: formerly the Hallervorden–Spatz Society; http://www.nbiadisorders.org. Caters for patients with NBIA.
- **International Parkinson and Movement Disorder Society**: http://www.movementdisorders.org.
- **EuroWilson**: European Reference Network for Wilson's Disease; http://www.eurowilson.org/.

# Chapter 10

# Drug-induced movement disorders

Introduction *250*
Drug-induced parkinsonism *252*
Drug-induced dystonia: 1 *254*
Drug-induced dystonia: 2 *256*
Drug-induced chorea *258*
Drug-induced tremor *260*
Drug-induced tics and myoclonus *262*
Other drug-induced movement disorder syndromes *264*

# Introduction

Drug-induced movement disorders are common. While drugs which affect dopamine transmission are the most frequent culprits, a range of other drugs with diverse modes of action can also cause drug-induced movement disorders.

### Clinical presentation of drug-induced movement disorders

There are two main presentations of drug-induced movement disorders:
- **Acute presentation:** rapid development of movement disorder following drug initiation
- **Tardive presentation:** gradual onset of movement disorder some time (often years) following drug initiation. This is a typical presentation of movement disorder due to DRBs. Despite drug withdrawal, the movement disorder will often continue.

### Common pitfalls in drug-induced movement disorders

It is not enough to simply ask the patient, where a drug-induced movement disorder is suspected, 'Have you started any new drugs recently?'. This will not identify all the patients where drugs may be the cause of the movement disorder for a number of reasons.
- **Dose increases of established drugs:** patients can develop a drug-induced movement disorder because of an increase in dose of an established medication. This may be missed if the patient is not asked about changes in *dose* of existing medication prior to the onset of the movement disorder.
- **Factors that alter plasma levels of established drugs:** patients can develop a drug-induced movement disorder caused by established drugs because of factors that can change plasma levels of medications. These factors include renal/liver failure and co-administration of drugs (e.g. co-administration of lamotrigine increases the plasma level of sodium valproate).
- **Patients do not consider all medications as 'drugs':** if patients are asked 'What medicines do you take?', they may not mention certain drugs, as they do not consider them to be medications. This is commonly the case for the oral contraceptive pill, herbal remedies, and nutritional supplements.
- **Drugs of abuse can cause movement disorders:** patients may not volunteer information about illicit drugs, unless directly asked. Nicotine and alcohol can also cause movement disorders and may not be mentioned by the patient.
- **Not all DRBs are antipsychotics:** DRBs which cause acute and tardive movement disorders are mainly used to treat psychosis. Patients treated for psychiatric problems with these drugs in the past may be reluctant to discuss this because of the stigma of mental illness. DRBs are also used to treat anxiety, nausea, and dizziness. A DRB that the patient is no longer taking may be the cause of the movement disorder.

### Important questions when considering a drug-induced movement disorder

- When did the movement disorder start in relationship to the commencement of any new medications?
- Was there a change in dose of an established medication prior to the onset of the movement disorder?
- Are there any factors that might have increased the plasma levels of established medications prior to the onset of the movement disorder?
- Specifically ask about exposure to DRBs at any point prior to the onset of movement disorder, including use of such drugs to treat nausea or dizziness.
- Specifically ask about exposure to:
  - oral contraceptive pill
  - illicit drugs
  - alcohol
  - nicotine
  - caffeine
  - 'over-the-counter' medications
  - Herbal remedies/nutritional supplements.

# Drug-induced parkinsonism

## Dopamine receptor-blocking drugs
DRBs are the commonest cause of drug-induced parkinsonism. Parkinsonism due to DRBs tends to be dose-related and is commoner with older antipsychotic drugs than with the newer 'atypical' antipsychotics. There are two main scenarios in which DRBs cause parkinsonism:
- patients with intact dopaminergic systems
- patients with underlying asymptomatic PD.

Surprisingly, clinical presentation can be very similar in both scenarios. Patients will have bradykinesia and rigidity, and often have resting tremor and a parkinsonian gait. Patients with underlying PD will tend to have asymmetric signs, but these can also occur in patients with intact dopaminergic systems.

### Investigation
With a clear history of DRB exposure in a young patient, investigation is often unnecessary. A DAT scan can be useful to differentiate between patients with pure drug-induced parkinsonism and patients with underlying PD. DRBs cause post-synaptic dopamine blockade, and therefore a DAT scan will be normal in pure drug-induced parkinsonism. Recently, large case series on patients with schizophrenia chronically treated with antipsychotics have shown that DAT scans may also be abnormal in such cases. However, clinico-pathological studies to exclude coexistent Lewy body pathology are missing.

### Management
If possible, the DRB should be stopped. This usually leads to resolution of symptoms within several weeks, but sometimes this may take as long as 3–6 months.

It may be impossible to stop DRB therapy, e.g. in patients with psychosis. If DRB therapy cannot be stopped, then the lowest dose necessary should be used, and the DRB switched to an 'atypical' DRB. Occasionally, use of levodopa can produce benefit in patients unable to stop or reduce the dose of their medication, but this is mostly seen in patients with underlying PD which has been revealed/worsened by DRB use.

### Tardive parkinsonism
A syndrome of parkinsonism which occurs after long-term DRB treatment and persists after DRB withdrawal has been described. It seems likely that this syndrome represents patients who have developed incidental PD. Their symptoms are revealed by DRB therapy and then remain present after DRB withdrawal because of continued progression of PD.

## Other drugs
Other drugs associated with parkinsonism are listed in Box 10.1.

## Box 10.1 Drugs associated with parkinsonism

### Dopamine receptor-blocking drugs

*'Older' antipsychotics*
- Chlorpromazine
- Haloperidol
- Flupentixol
- Sulpiride
- Pimozide
- Trifluoperazine

*'Atypical' antipsychotics*
- Quetiapine
- Clozapine
- Risperidone
- Olanzapine
- Amisulpride
- Sertindole
- Zotepine

*Others*
- Metoclopramide
- Prochlorperazine

### Dopamine-depleting drugs
- Tetrabenazine

### Other drugs
- Cinnarizine
- Fluphenazine
- Lithium
- Amiodarone
- Sodium valproate
- Diltiazem

# Drug-induced dystonia: 1

Once again, the commonest drugs causing dystonia are DRBs. ADRs are seen with DRBs, as well as many other prescribed drugs and drugs of abuse. Tardive dystonia occurs only with chronic exposure to DRBs.

## Acute dystonic reactions

- ADRs usually occur in the period shortly after administration of a drug, most commonly a DRB.
- About 2% of those beginning treatment with a DRB will develop an ADR.
- Time to onset is variable, but 50% will show symptoms within 2 days, and 90% will have done so within 5 days.
- Common presentations are with oromandibular dystonia, oculogyric crisis (conjugate deviation of the eyes, usually accompanied by facial dystonia and sometimes psychotic features such as hallucinations and obsessional thoughts), hyperextension of the spine and/or neck, and laryngeal dystonic spasm.
- Apart from DRBs, a number of other prescription drugs and drugs of abuse with diverse modes of action can cause ADRs (Box 10.2).
- Levodopa can cause ADRs in the context of PD: peak-dose and off-period dystonia (→ p. 73). Patients with MSA exposed to levodopa can develop an acute facial dystonia (dystonic grimace; → p. 102).
- Treatment can be an emergency because of respiratory compromise and is primarily with anticholinergic drugs.

### Treatment of acute dystonic reactions

- Basic life support assessment: airways, breathing, circulation.
- Basic supportive treatment for any compromise (e.g. oxygen, monitor oxygen saturations, consider need for intubation).
- Benzatropine 1–2 mg IV, or procyclidine 5–10 mg IV. Usually effective over 5–10 minutes.
- Main side effects: dry mouth, hallucinations, confusion. Contraindicated in closed-angle glaucoma and gastrointestinal obstruction.
- If failure to respond, reconsider the diagnosis; repeat injection of benzatropine/procyclidine; give clonazepam 1–2 mg (main side effect: sedation and respiratory depression).
- Start oral trihexyphenidyl 2 mg tds for 2–5 days to prevent recurrence.
- Stop the offending drug.
- Continue to monitor for 24 hours in hospital in case of recurrence.

### Box 10.2 Commonly reported causes of acute dystonic reactions

- Dopamine receptor-blocking drugs
- Amine depletors (e.g. tetrabenazine)
- Antidepressants: serotonin reuptake inhibitors, monoamine oxidase inhibitors
- Calcium antagonists
- Benzodiazepines
- General anaesthetic agents
- Anticonvulsants (carbamazepine, phenytoin)
- Triptans
- Ranitidine
- Cocaine
- Ecstasy

# Drug-induced dystonia: 2

### Tardive dystonia and tardive dyskinesia

*Clinical features*
- Tardive dystonia and tardive dyskinesia are overlapping clinical syndromes caused by chronic exposure to DRBs (see Video 10.1: Tardive dystonia).
- In **tardive dyskinesia**, the characteristic features are of choreiform movements around the mouth and lower face, resulting in characteristic lip smacking and tongue writhing movements. The limbs and trunk may also be affected.
- In **tardive dystonia**, the characteristic features are of axial dystonia with hyperextension of the spine and retrocollis.
- Tardive dyskinesia is commoner in older patients exposed to DRB, while tardive dystonia is commoner in younger patients. Many patients will have elements of both dystonia and chorea.

*Causes*
- All DRBs appear to be capable of producing tardive dyskinsia/ dystonia, although it is less common with the 'atypical' DRBs. Amine depletors (e.g. tetrabenazine) do not cause tardive syndromes.
- Tardive dyskinesia/dystonia usually occurs after prolonged exposure to DRBs (mean time from exposure to onset 6 years), but the shortest exposure time to onset reported is 4 days.
- The pathophysiology of tardive syndromes is unknown but may relate to receptor hypersensitivity caused by chronic receptor blockade.

*Treatment*
- Prevention is clearly the best option by only using a DRB (preferably an atypical DRB) when necessary and for as short a period as possible.
- If tardive syndromes do occur, spontaneous remission occurs in only 10% of patients. Remission is more likely with prompt discontinuation of the DRB when symptoms occur and with a shorter total duration of exposure to DRB.
- First-line treatment of tardive dystonia is with anticholinergic drugs such as trihexyphenidyl. Other drugs that can be tried include benzodiazepines, baclofen, and tetrabenazine, but little evidence exists to support their use. For tardive chorea, tetrabenazine is a first-line therapy.
- BT injections can be helpful for tardive dystonia affecting the neck. Intrathecal baclofen has been used in some patients with severe axial dystonia, with reported good results in some.
- DBS of the GPi has been used in tardive dystonia and may be of excellent benefit in some patients.
- Paradoxically, reintroduction of certain DRBs can lead to an improvement in symptoms in patients with refractory tardive dyskinesia/dystonia. Clozapine has some controlled trial evidence to support its use in this situation (but requires blood monitoring; see Box 10.3). Other 'atypical' DRBs, such as olanzapine, risperidone, and quetiapine, have also been used, with reported success.

### Box 10.3 How to introduce medications commonly used for the treatment of tardive dystonia/dyskinesia

#### Trihexyphenidyl (benzhexol)

- Available as generic tablets in 2 mg and 5 mg tablets (white, scored) or in syrup (5 mg/5 mL).
- Starting dose is 1 mg daily.
- Increase by 1 mg every 4–7 days to reach 1 mg tds. Then increase by 1 mg every 4–7 days to reach 2–4 mg tds.
- If side effects occur, dose titration should be stopped and then re-attempted after 1–2 weeks. Maximum dose may be as high as 50–100 mg daily.*
- Common side effects: dry mouth, dry eyes, nausea, confusion, constipation, urinary retention.
- Important contraindication: closed-angle glaucoma.

#### Tetrabenazine

- Available in 25 mg tablets (yellow-buff, scored).
- Starting dose is 12.5 mg once daily.
- Increase every week by 12.5 mg to reach 12.5 mg tds, and then increase in 12.5 mg increments to reach 25–50 mg tds as symptoms require.
- Maximum dose 200 mg daily.
- Main side effects are parkinsonism and depression.

#### Clonazepam

- Available in 500 micrograms (beige) or 2 mg (white) tablets (scored twice).
- Starting dose is 250 micrograms once daily (125 micrograms in the elderly).
- Increase every week by 250 micrograms to reach 500 micrograms to 1 mg bd to tds.
- Maximum dose 4–6 mg daily.
- Main side effects are sedation, depression, and fatigue.

#### Clozapine

- Available in 25 mg and 100 mg tablets.
- Clozapine causes agranulocytosis, and all patients must be registered with a clozapine blood monitoring programme which is organized by the pharmaceutical companies that manufacture the product. Clozapine also causes myocarditis and cardiomyopathy; therefore it is relatively contraindicated in those with a history of cardiac disease. Physical examination to exclude signs of cardiac disease is required prior to drug initiation.
- Typical starting dose is 12.5 mg daily, with a typical maintenance dose of 25–50 mg daily in two divided doses.
- Prescription of clozapine should ideally be done in cooperation with a psychiatrist familiar with the medication and the monitoring programmes.

# Drug-induced chorea

The two most important causes of drug-induced chorea are discussed elsewhere:
- levodopa-induced dyskinesia (chorea) in PD (➔ p. 73)
- tardive dyskinesia (chorea) due to chronic DRB exposure.

Other causes of drug-induced chorea are given in Box 10.4. An important pitfall to be aware of is that anticholinergic drugs, such as trihexyphenidyl, can cause chorea. This can create diagnostic confusion when anticholinergics are used to treat patients with dystonia. If such patients then develop chorea, it can be difficult to determine whether the chorea is caused by the anticholinergic drug or is part of the underlying movement disorder.

### Box 10.4 Drugs associated with chorea
- Chronic levodopa treatment in Parkinson's disease
- Chronic dopamine receptor-blocking drug treatment
- Oral contraceptives
- Anticholinergics (e.g. trihexyphenidyl)
- Anticonvulsants (e.g. phenytoin)
- Thyroxine
- Benzodiazepines
- Monoamine oxidase inhibitors
- Tricyclic antidepressants (e.g. amitriptyline)
- Digoxin
- Alcohol withdrawal

# Drug-induced tremor

Tremor is a side effect of treatment with a wide range of drugs. Drug-induced tremor is usually postural, and, when a rest tremor occurs, this is usually in the context of drug-induced parkinsonism (➜ p. 252). Box 10.5 gives a list of the commonest drugs causing tremor. Freely available drugs, such as coffee, nicotine, and alcohol, and drugs of abuse, such as cocaine and marijuana, can also cause tremor.

'Tardive tremor' is a rare entity, reported to occur after chronic use of DRBs and continuing after the DRBs have been withdrawn. As is the case with tardive parkinsonism, there is debate as to whether this syndrome does indeed exist or really reflects underlying PD.

### Box 10.5 Drugs associated with tremor

#### Drugs which may cause tremor (usually resting) and parkinsonism
- Dopamine receptor-blocking drugs
- Dopamine-depleting drugs
- Calcium channel-blocking drugs
- Lithium
- Amiodarone
- Sodium valproate

#### Drugs which commonly cause tremor (usually postural)
- Beta-agonists (e.g. salbutamol)
- Anticonvulsants (e.g. sodium valproate)
- Thyroxine
- Tricyclic antidepressants
- Theophylline
- Lithium
- Immunosuppressive drugs (e.g. ciclosporin)
- Alcohol
- Caffeine
- Nicotine
- Mercury
- Drugs of abuse (e.g. marijuana, cocaine, amphetamines)

# Drug-induced tics and myoclonus

## Drug-induced tics
Drugs commonly associated with tics are listed in Box 10.6. Most important amongst these are amphetamines, which tend to cause tics after chronic use. Methylphenidate, which is used for the treatment of ADHD, may worsen tics, but this is not always the case. This is important to note, as ADHD often accompanies TS, and methylphenidate may be prescribed (➔ p. 153).

A tardive tic syndrome has been described after chronic use of DRBs and persisting after their withdrawal. As with tardive parkinsonism and tremor, this is not a certain clinical entity.

## Drug-induced myoclonus
Box 10.7 gives a list of the commonest drugs associated with myoclonus. Drug toxicity commonly leads to myoclonus. This need not occur simply due to overdose. It can occur when metabolism of a particular drug is impaired in hepatic or renal failure.

### Box 10.6 Drugs associated with tics or that can worsen pre-existing tic disorder
- Methylphenidate
- Amantadine
- Fenfluramine
- Levodopa
- Carbamazepine
- Drugs of abuse, including cocaine, ecstasy, amphetamines

### Box 10.7 Drugs commonly associated with myoclonus
- Levodopa
- Benzodiazepines
- Opioid analgesics
- Anticonvulsants (in particular, gabapentin, pregabalin, phenytoin, valproate, lamotrigine, and phenobarbital)
- Tricyclic antidepressants
- Bismuth salts
- Anaesthetic agents
- Selective serotonin reuptake inhibitors

# Other drug-induced movement disorder syndromes

### Neuroleptic malignant syndrome
- Neuroleptic malignant syndrome (NMS) is a medical emergency characterized by rigidity, high fever, hypertension, excessive sweating, and fluctuating level of consciousness.
- It is an iatrogenic syndrome associated with DRB use, usually within 2 weeks of starting treatment or if doses of existing DRBs are being escalated.
- An NMS-like syndrome can also occur in patients with PD if their dopaminergic drugs are suddenly stopped.
- NMS can be fatal, and early treatment is essential. There are no diagnostic tests, and a high clinical index of suspicion is needed. Usually a raised CK and white cell count will be found. CSF studies and brain imaging are usually normal.

### Treatment of neuroleptic malignant syndrome
- Adequate supportive care is a key feature of successful treatment, and patients with NMS should be managed in a high-dependency unit (HDU) or intensive care unit (ICU) setting.
- Control of blood pressure, temperature, and electrolyte balance is important, as well as monitoring for signs of rhabdomyolysis and consequent renal failure.
- The DRB should be withdrawn.
- Treatment is with IV dantrolene sodium, starting at a dose of 2–3 mg/kg/day in three divided doses, rising to a maximum of 10 mg/kg/day if required. Dantrolene acts as a muscle relaxant by preventing the release of calcium from stores within muscle.
- Give dopamine agonists orally or via a nasogastric tube (e.g. ropinirole 5 mg tds or pramipexole 1 mg tds). An apomorphine infusion or administration of a rotigotine patch 16mg daily can be used in patients where oral or nasogastric access is not possible.

### Neuroleptic malignant syndrome-like syndromes
Parkinsonism–hyperpyrexia syndrome (PHS), akinetic crisis (AC), dyskinesia–hyperpyrexia syndrome, and serotonin syndrome (SS) share similarities with NMS clinically and therefore lie under the umbrella of NMS-like syndromes.

#### Parkinsonism–hyperpyrexia syndrome and akinetic crisis
- These conditions are usually due to withdrawal from levodopa or other dopaminergic drugs such as dopamine agonists, amantadine, or COMT inhibitors. PHS has also been reported after STN DBS or withdrawal from STN DBS.
- The clinical picture is quite similar to NMS.

- Further complications include aspiration pneumonia, deep venous thrombosis, pulmonary thromboembolism, disseminated intravascular coagulation, rhabdomyolysis, acute renal failure, seizures, and respiratory failure.
- Mortality rates are high (4–12%).
- Roughly two-thirds of patients with PHS will recover following adequate management.

### Serotonin syndrome

- SS results from exposure to drugs increasing serotonin activity, including SSRIs, serotonin and noradrenaline reuptake inhibitors (SNRIs), tricyclics, monoamine oxidase inhibitors (MAOIs), lithium, opiates, and antiepileptics.
- SS develops as an acute condition within 24 hours after drug initiation, sometimes only a few hours, with 60% of cases within the first 6 hours.
- SS can present with subtle and non-specific symptoms to lethal multiorgan failure.
- Typical manifestations include an altered mental state characterized by agitation, anxiety, confusion, or euphoria, dysautonomia with fever, tachycardia, high blood pressure, tachypnoea, diaphoresis, and diarrhoea, and various movements disorders such as tremor, akathisia, and, more notably, myoclonus.
- Additional neurological abnormalities can be found, including mydriasis, rigidity, hyperreflexia, clonus, and altered coordination, usually more marked in the lower limbs.
- Treatment requires immediate discontinuation of the offending agent which may be sufficient to achieve complete recovery within 24 hours.
- ICU when required by severity of symptoms, benzodiazepines, or 5-HT2A receptor antagonists such as cryptoheptadine, chlorpromazine, or olanzapine.

## Akathisia

- Akathisia is a feeling of inner restlessness and a desire to move, accompanied by the physical expression of this feeling.
- This physical expression can range from small movements, such as drumming of the fingers or shifting position, to a necessity to walk or even run.
- It is most commonly caused by DRB use. It has also been described as a tardive syndrome following chronic DRB exposure. Treatment is with reduction of DRB dose or withdrawal, if possible, and with anticholinergics such as procyclidine and trihexyphenidyl, and benzodiazepines.
- Akathisia has also been reported to occur with serotonin reuptake inhibitors, antihistamines, and tricyclic antidepressants.
- Akathisia can be difficult to differentiate from RLS (→ p. 294). In contrast to RLS, akathisia tends to occur all day, rather than just in the evening, and is associated with an urge to move, but not necessarily dictated by uncomfortable sensations in the legs.

### Withdrawal emergent syndrome

This syndrome is described predominantly in children following sudden withdrawal of chronic DRB therapy. Generalized chorea, which can be very severe, occurs and typically remits over several days or weeks. Treatment is supportive, and, if severe, the DRB may be reintroduced and then withdrawn more slowly at a later date.

### Dopamine agonist withdrawal syndrome (DAWS)

Recently, patients have been reported who have developed a neuropsychiatric syndrome characterized by agitation, depression, autonomic symptoms (postural dizziness, sweating), fatigue, and insomnia on withdrawal from dopamine agonist medication. Most reported patients were withdrawn from the drugs due to the presence of impulse control disorders in the context of treatment for PD. However, case reports of a similar syndrome exist for patients without PD, e.g. patients receiving dopamine agonists for RLS and a pituitary tumour. Use of levodopa does not seem to help symptoms. Most patients experience a gradual reduction of symptoms over weeks to months, but, for some with persistent symptoms, re-prescription of the dopamine agonist is suggested (if possible), followed by slow withdrawal.

# Chapter 11

# Paroxysmal movement disorders

Introduction 268
Paroxysmal dyskinesia: 1 270
Paroxysmal dyskinesia: 2 272
Episodic ataxias 276

# Introduction

The paroxysmal movement disorders are a rare group of conditions characterized by episodes of abnormal movement that are self-limiting. Most paroxysmal movement disorders are 'primary', i.e. occur without a secondary cause, and are not part of a neurodegenerative process. In these cases, patients are usually symptom-free between attacks, and autosomal dominant inheritance is often seen. Occasionally, paroxysmal movement disorders occur as secondary phenomena, e.g. as a result of perinatal brain injury or with PD. Such patients will usually have additional neurological symptoms and signs that are persistent between attacks.

## Classification

Paroxysmal movement disorders are divided into two groups:
- paroxysmal dyskinesia: attacks are usually a mixture of chorea and dystonia (Table 11.1)
- episodic ataxias: attacks of ataxia (Table 11.2).

Clinical classification is then based on:
- the length of the attack
- the precipitants of an attack.

## Pathophysiology

Many paroxysmal movement disorders are thought to be *channelopathies*, i.e. abnormalities of the control of cellular entry or exit of ions such as calcium or potassium. It is possible that these abnormalities in ion flux cause changes in the excitability of neurons within the basal ganglia which, if a certain threshold is reached, can lead to a transient impairment of motor control and the production of abnormal movement.

## Treatment

Some paroxysmal movement disorders are easily treatable. As would be expected from the pathophysiology of these disorders, the medications that are effective, such as carbamazepine and acetazolamide, act on ion channels.

### Types of paroxysmal movement disorders

*Paroxysmal dyskinesia*
- Paroxysmal kinesigenic dyskinesia (PKD)
- Paroxysmal non-kinesigenic dyskinesia (PNKD)
- Paroxysmal exercise-induced dyskinesia (PED)
- Paroxysmal nocturnal dyskinesia (PND)

*Episodic ataxias*
- Episodic ataxia type 1 (EA1)
- Episodic ataxia type 2 (EA2)

# Paroxysmal dyskinesia: 1

## Paroxysmal kinesigenic dyskinesia

### Clinical features
- Characterized by *brief* attacks (seconds to minutes) of chorea and dystonia precipitated by *sudden movement* (see Video 11.1: PKD).
- A typical story is that attacks occur following a sudden unexpected movement (such as jumping up to answer the telephone).
- A typical attack is of abnormal posturing or movement of a limb. Attacks usually affect just one side of the body, but generalized attacks also occur.
- Sometimes hundreds of attacks may occur per day.
- Consciousness is fully preserved throughout an attack.

### Differential diagnosis
- *Epileptic* seizures, but paroxysmal kinesigenic dyskinesia (PKD) is kinesigenic, and consciousness is preserved.
- *Tonic spasms*, e.g. in multiple sclerosis, but these are painful.

### Aetiology and treatment
- PKD often occurs as a 'primary' phenomenon, with onset in childhood. Late onset (up to 50 years) has been reported. Patients are symptom-free between attacks.
- Autosomal dominant inheritance may be seen, and mutations in the proline-rich transmembrane protein 2 (*PRRT2*) gene have been identified as causative in many PKD families. The PRRT2 protein has been shown to interact with synaptosomal-associated protein 25 (SNAP25), suggesting a role in the fusion of synaptic vesicles to the plasma membrane.
- Mutations in *PRRT2* have been associated with a variety of further paroxysmal disorders that may or may not coexist in the same patient or in patients of the same family (Box 11.1).
- Primary PKD is typically exquisitely responsive to small doses of carbamazepine (100–200 mg/day). Attacks usually lessen with age. Other treatment options include phenytoin and acetazolamide.
- PKD can occur secondary to brain injury (e.g. perinatal hypoxia), in which case patients usually have other neurological signs.

### Box 11.1 PRRT2-associated paroxysmal conditions
- Classic paroxysmal kinesigenic dyskinesia
- Infantile convulsions with paroxysmal choreoathetosis (ICCA)
- Benign familial infantile epilepsy
- Migraine with or without aura
- Hemiplegic migraine
- Episodic ataxia
- Paroxysmal exercise-induced dyskinesia (PED) (rarely)
- Paroxysmal non-kinesigenic dyskinesia (PNKD) (rarely)

## Paroxysmal non-kinesigenic dyskinesia

- Characterized by more prolonged attacks (minutes to hours) of chorea and dystonia precipitated by coffee, alcohol, and fatigue. Onset is usually in childhood (see Video 11.2: PNKD).
- Attacks are usually generalized but may be focal. Between attacks, patients are symptom-free.
- A maximum of two or three attacks will occur per day. Typically, only a few attacks occur per year.
- Treatment is difficult. Precipitants should be avoided. There is a limited response to phenytoin, acetazolamide, benzodiazepines, and levodopa.
- Mutations in the myofibrillogenesis regulator 1 (*MR1*) gene have been reported in some families with autosomal dominant inheritance. The gene product plays a role in the detoxification of methylglyoxal, a compound present in coffee, alcoholic drinks, and formed as a by-product of oxidative stress. Rarely, *PRRT2* mutations have been described in patients that share more phenotypic features with paroxysmal non-kinesigenic dyskinesia (PNKD) than PKD.

Table 11.1 Clinical features of paroxysmal dyskinesias

| | Paroxysmal kinesigenic dyskinesia | Paroxysmal non-kinesigenic dyskinesia | Paroxysmal exercise-induced dyskinesia |
|---|---|---|---|
| Age at onset | Childhood/teens | Childhood/teens | Variable |
| Precipitating factors | Sudden movement | Coffee, alcohol, fatigue | Prolonged exertion |
| Nature of attacks | Chorea/dystonia | Chorea/dystonia | Dystonia |
| Length of attacks | Seconds to minutes | Minutes to hours | Subside with rest |
| Number of attacks per day | Up to hundreds per day | Up to 2–3 per day | Dependent on exercise |
| Treatment | Carbamazepine | Avoid precipitants. Treat with phenytoin, acetazolamide, benzodiazepines, levodopa | Avoid precipitants. Treat underlying cause |
| Aetiology | Familial cases due to PRRT2. Can be secondary to brain injury | Some familial cases due to mutations in myofibrillogenesis regulator gene | May be due to GLUT1 deficiency or secondary to parkinsonian disorders |

# Paroxysmal dyskinesia: 2

## Paroxysmal exercise-induced dystonia

### Clinical features
- Characterized by attacks of dystonia precipitated by prolonged exercise (📽 see Video 11.3: PED).
- Dystonia almost always affects the limb that has been exercised, although spread to adjacent muscles can be seen. The dystonia will emerge gradually as exercise continues and will increase in severity until exercise has stopped. With rest, there is typically a resolution of the dystonia over 1–2 minutes.

### Aetiology and treatment
- Paroxysmal exercise-induced dystonia (PED) can occur as a primary condition with an autosomal dominant inheritance. Onset is typically in childhood.
- Heterozygous mutations in the *SLC2A1* gene encoding for glucose transporter 1 (GLUT1) have been identified as causative for PED in many patients with familial and sporadic forms. GLUT1 is a major glucose transporter in the blood–brain barrier. Central hypoglycaemia in situations of greater energy demand can explain exercise and fasting as triggers in PED.
- *SLC2A1* mutations are associated with a wide phenotypic spectrum beyond PED (Box 11.2).
- Diagnosis can be made by lumbar puncture, showing low CSF glucose levels with normal lactate, a CSF glucose/plasma glucose ratio of <0.45, as well as by genetic testing.
- PED commonly occurs in conditions of dopamine depletion such as PD and DRD. Therefore, these diagnoses should be considered in patients with PED, particularly if there are additional neurological signs (e.g. bradykinesia) or a progressive history.
- PED has been reported as long as 5 years prior to the diagnosis of PD. A DAT scan can be helpful to look for evidence of pre-synaptic dopamine loss, as seen in PD. Tests for DRD (phenylalanine loading test, CSF pterins; ➲ p. 213) are appropriate in patients with young-onset PED.
- Treatment of primary PED includes avoidance of prolonged exercise and fasting. Moreover, in patients with PED due to GLUT1 mutations, a ketogenic diet may be of benefit. It is a high-fat, carbohydrate-restricted diet that mimics the metabolic state of fasting and provides an alternative fuel source for the brain (ketone bodies).
- PED secondary to PD or DRD can be successfully treated by dopaminergic treatment.

### Box 11.2 GLUT1 deficiency syndromes
- Epileptic encephalopathy with complex movement disorders, mental retardation, microcephaly, and very early onset (<1 year)
- Early-onset absence epilepsy (EOAE) (<4 years)
- Classic idiopathic generalized epilepsies, including childhood absence epilepsy (CAE)
- Seizures and episodic ataxia
- Classic paroxysmal exercise-induced dystonia
- Alternating hemiplegia

### Paroxysmal nocturnal dyskinesia
- This is a heterogeneous entity characterized by attacks of abnormal posturing during sleep.
- Causes include the following:
  - frontal lobe epilepsy, in particular autosomal dominant nocturnal frontal lobe epilepsy (ADNFLE). This is a dominantly inherited childhood-onset epilepsy syndrome with predominantly nocturnal seizures. About 20–30% of patients have mutations in genes encoding subunits of the nicotinic acetylcholine receptor (*CHNRA4, CHNRB2*). Testing for these mutations is available as a clinical service
  - RBD (→ p. 298)
  - PLMS (→ p. 295)
  - 'off-period' dystonia in PD (→ p. 73).
- Polysomnography with video and EEG recording can be a helpful investigation.

### How to introduce medications commonly used for the treatment of paroxysmal dyskinesia

*Carbamazepine*
- Available in generic form in 100 mg, 200 mg, and 400 mg tablets.
- Starting dose 100 mg daily.
- Wait 2–3 weeks to monitor effect.
- If insufficient benefits, increase to 100 mg bd, and consider further increases in 100 mg increments every 2–3 weeks as required.
- Maximum dose: 1.6–2 g daily, but most patients with PKD will need much less (200–400 mg). If symptoms are not controlled on moderate doses, reconsider the diagnosis.
- Common side effects: nausea, vomiting, diplopia, raised liver enzymes, hyponatraemia. Rarely causes agranulocytosis and rash.
- Carbamazepine induces liver enzymes and therefore interferes with the effectiveness of many drugs, including *warfarin* and the *oral contraceptive pill*.

*Acetazolamide*
- Available in 250 mg tablets.
- Start at 250 mg daily.
- Increase dose, if necessary, after 2–3 weeks in 250 mg increments to reach 250 mg bd or tds.
- Maximum dose: 1 g daily.
- Common side effects: nausea, vomiting, paraesthesiae in fingers and toes, headache. In long-term use, agranulocytosis and electrolyte disturbance may occur. Prolonged treatment requires periodic monitoring of electrolytes.

*Phenytoin*
- Available as generic tablets 25 mg, 50 mg, 100 mg, and 300 mg capsules.
- Start at 50 mg daily.
- Increase dose, if necessary, after 2–3 weeks in 50 mg increments to reach 150–300 mg once daily.
- Maximum dose: dependent on plasma levels—in the region of 400–500 mg daily.
- Main side effects: sedation, nausea, ataxia, confusion. Stevens–Johnson syndrome can occur.
- Phenytoin has zero-order kinetics, and therefore a small increase in dose can lead to a large increase in plasma levels.

# Episodic ataxias

## Episodic ataxia type 1 (EA1)
- Characterized by brief episodes of ataxia (seconds to minutes) precipitated by sudden movement or startle.
- Onset is typically in childhood, and many attacks occur per day.
- Between attacks, some patients have *myokymia* (rapid twitching due to activation of single muscle fibres) and *neuromyotonia* (continuous motor unit activity causing muscle contraction and cramping). Both myokymia and neuromyotonia have typical appearances on EMG.
- The condition has autosomal dominant inheritance and is due to mutations in a potassium channel gene (*KCNA1*).
- Treatment with acetazolamide is often very effective. Phenytoin is also effective in some patients.

## Episodic ataxia type 2 (EA2)
- Characterized by prolonged episodes of ataxia (hours to days) precipitated by coffee, alcohol, and fatigue.
- Onset is typically in childhood or teenage years. Only up to one or two attacks will occur per day, and often only a few attacks per year.
- During attacks, patients may experience vertigo, nausea, and fever.
- Between attacks, patients are initially symptom-free, but, over time, many patients develop progressive ataxia and nystagmus.
- EA2 is inherited in an autosomal dominant fashion and is due to mutations in a calcium channel gene on chromosome 19p (*CACNA1A*).
- This gene is also mutated in SCA 6 (CAG repeat expansions) and in familial hemiplegic migraine 1 (FHM1) (nonsense and missense mutations). Moreover, *CACNA1A* mutations are associated with benign paroxysmal torticollis in children and paroxysmal tonic upgaze of infancy.
- A phenotypically similar condition episodic ataxia type 5 (EA5) is due to mutations in a different calcium channel gene on chromosome 2q (*CACNB4B4*).
- Treatment is less successful than in EA1, but acetazolamide may be effective.

**Table 11.2** Clinical features of episodic ataxia

|  | Episodic ataxia type 1 | Episodic ataxia type 2 |
| --- | --- | --- |
| Age at onset | Childhood/teens | Childhood/teens |
| Precipitating factors | Sudden movement | Coffee, alcohol, fatigue |
| Nature of attacks | Ataxia | Ataxia ± nausea, vertigo, and fever |
| Length of attacks | Seconds to minutes | Hours to days |
| Number of attacks per day | Hundreds per day | Up to two or three per day |
| Other features | Interictal myokymia and neuromyotonia | Progressive interictal ataxia and nystagmus |
| Treatment | Acetazolamide, phenytoin | Acetazolamide |
| Aetiology | *KCNA1* gene mutations | *CACNA1A* gene mutations (*CACNB4B4* mutations cause a phenotypically similar condition—episodic ataxia type 5) |

# Chapter 12

# Movement disorders and ataxia

Introduction *280*
Inherited ataxia and movement disorders *282*
Fragile X-associated tremor/ataxia syndrome *286*
Other causes of movement disorder and ataxia *288*
Useful websites and addresses *290*

# Introduction

This chapter does not explore the differential diagnosis of ataxia in general. Instead, it concentrates on those disorders where cerebellar signs and movement disorders occur together.

### An approach to movement disorders and ataxia

Table 12.1 lists conditions where movement disorders and ataxia occur together. The presentation of these disorders is often highly variable. Within a group of patients with the same condition, some may have cerebellar signs without a movement disorder, while, in others, the movement disorder may be the dominant feature. A mixture of movement disorders often occurs. These features make the differential diagnosis of these disorders quite difficult.

Many of the conditions causing ataxia and movement disorders are discussed in other chapters, as indicated in Table 12.1.

# INTRODUCTION

**Table 12.1** Cerebellar syndromes and different movement disorders

| | |
|---|---|
| Cerebellar syndrome and parkinsonism (including rest tremor) | Multiple system atrophy (→ p. 102)<br>Spinocerebellar ataxia (SCA) 1, 2, 3, 7, 17 (in particular SCA 2, 3)<br>Fragile X pre-mutation carriers (FXTAS)<br>Wilson's disease (→ p. 220) |
| Cerebellar syndrome and tremor (typically postural tremor) | SCA 6, 12, 27 (SCA 16—head tremor)<br>Friedreich's ataxia<br>Multiple sclerosis<br>Brainstem lesions<br>Fragile X pre-mutation carriers (FXTAS)<br>Wilson's disease (→ p. 220) |
| Cerebellar syndrome and chorea | SCA 1, 2, 3, 7, 17<br>Huntington's disease (→ p. 164)<br>Wilson's disease (→ p. 220)<br>Ataxia telangiectasia<br>Friedreich's ataxia<br>Coeliac disease<br>Dentatorubropallidoluysian atrophy (DRPLA) (→ p. 187)<br>Ataxia with oculomotor apraxia 1 and 2 |
| Cerebellar syndrome and myoclonus | SCA 2, 14, 19<br>Unverricht–Lundborg disease (→ p. 186)<br>Sialidosis (→ p. 186)<br>Neuronal ceroid lipofuscinosis (→ p. 186)<br>Lafora body disease (→ p. 186)<br>Mitochondrial disease (→ p. 186)<br>DRPLA (→ p. 187)<br>Progressive ataxia palatal tremor syndrome (PAPT)<br>Coeliac disease<br>Multiple system atrophy (→ p. 102)<br>Creutzfeldt–Jakob disease<br>Paraneoplastic (opsoclonus–myoclonus) |
| Cerebellar syndrome and dystonia | SCA 1, 2, 3, 7, 14, 17<br>Wilson's disease (→ p. 220)<br>Ataxia telangiectasia<br>Friedreich's ataxia<br>Fragile X pre-mutation carriers (FXTAS)<br>DRPLA (→ p. 187)<br>Multiple system atrophy (→ p. 102)<br>Cervical dystonia and progressive ataxia syndrome<br>Ataxia with oculomotor apraxia 1 and 2<br>Niemann–Pick type C<br>GLUT1 mutation carriers |

# Inherited ataxia and movement disorders

## Dominant ataxia syndromes: spinocerebellar ataxia

The SCAs are a group of inherited degenerative conditions primarily affecting the cerebellum. SCAs are almost all dominantly inherited, and many are caused by triplet repeat expansions. All cause a progressive cerebellar syndrome, but, in some cases, movement disorders also occur. Rarely, movement disorders are the dominant clinical feature of the condition.

### Clinical features

Table 12.2 gives a brief summary of the clinical features of the main SCAs associated with movement disorders in order to guide recognition and appropriate genetic testing.

Table 12.2

| SCA | Onset age | Clinical features |
|---|---|---|
| 1 | Forties | Ataxia, ophthalmoplegia, dystonia, chorea, neuropathy, pyramidal signs, mild dementia. Particularly common in South Africa |
| 2 | Variable: usually <25 years | Ataxia, ophthalmoplegia (very slow horizontal saccades), pyramidal signs, neuropathy, parkinsonism (may be levodopa-responsive), myoclonus, tremor, dystonia |
| 3 | Variable: twenties to forties | Very variable. May include ataxia, ophthalmoplegia, parkinsonism (may be levodopa-responsive), dystonia, chorea, spasticity. Particularly common in South America |
| 6 | Variable: most >50 years | Ataxia with postural tremor. May mimic essential tremor, rarely parkinsonism has also been described |
| 7 | Most <20 years | Ataxia, retinal degeneration, neuropathy, rarely chorea |
| 12 | Forties | Ataxia with postural tremor. May mimic essential tremor |
| 14 | Thirties | Ataxia with myoclonus, tremor, and rarely dystonia. Mild neuropathy |
| 16 | Forties | Japanese family with ataxia and head tremor |
| 17 | Forties or later | May present with parkinsonism and later with chorea, also ataxia and cognitive impairment |
| 19 | 20–45 years | Dutch family with mild ataxia, myoclonus, postural tremor, cognitive decline, mild neuropathy |
| 27 | Teens | Dutch family with ataxia, tremor, orofacial dyskinesia, and cognitive decline |
| DRPLA | Teens to sixties | Ataxia, myoclonus, epilepsy, chorea, dystonia, cognitive decline. Very rare in most populations, but particularly common in Japan where it is commoner than Huntington's disease. Homozygotes with intermediate number of repeats may have spastic paraparesis and truncal ataxia. DRPLA is allelic to the Haw River syndrome—progressive dementia associated with demyelination |

### Recessive ataxia syndromes associated with movement disorders

Table 12.3 shows some recessive ataxia syndromes associated with movement disorders. A number of inherited ataxia conditions are covered elsewhere: progressive myoclonic epilepsy ataxia syndromes (➔ p. 186), WD (➔ p. 220), and AT.

- **Friedreich's ataxia**: a common cause of autosomal recessive progressive ataxia due to mutations in the frataxin gene. Mean age at onset is 14 years, but late onset is seen. Clinical features include ataxia, pyramidal signs, sensorimotor neuropathy, and optic atrophy. Rare patients have been reported presenting with chorea without ataxia. MRI may show no or minimal atrophy of the cerebellum, but instead atrophy of the cervical cord.
- **Ataxia and oculomotor apraxia type 1 (AOA1)**: an autosomal recessive disorder of childhood onset (mean age 5 years), combining ataxia, oculomotor apraxia (problem mainly with horizontal eye movements—the child has to use head thrusts to defixate/fixate), dystonia, chorea, parkinsonism, sensorimotor neuropathy, due to mutations in the aprataxin gene.
- **Ataxia and oculomotor apraxia type 2 (AOA2)**: an autosomal recessive disorder of teenage onset (mean age 15 years, can present in early adult life). Clinical features are similar to AOA1, due to mutations in the senataxin gene.

Finally, there are some recessive ataxias that can be treatable and therefore should not be missed. These include Niemann–Pick type C, cerebrotendinous xanthomatosis, abetalipoproteinaemia, Refsum's disease, and ataxia with coenzyme Q10 deficiency.

Table 12.3 Clinical features of recessive ataxias associated with movement disorders

| Disease (gene) | Phenotype | Age at onset (years) |
|---|---|---|
| Friedreich's ataxia (FRDA) | Mixed cerebellar/sensory ataxia, areflexia, pyramidal weakness, extensor plantar responses. Chorea, tremor, and dystonia have been described | 5–25 Late-onset possible |
| Hereditary ataxia with vitamin E deficiency (TTPA) | Like Friedreich's, visual loss or retinitis pigmentosa, chorea | <20 |
| Refsum's disease (PHYH) | Polyneuropathy, sensorineural deafness, retinitis pigmentosa, anosmia | <20 Late-onset possible |
| Abetalipoproteinaemia (MTP) | Like Friedreich's, retinitis pigmentosa, malabsorption | <20 |
| Autosomal recessive spastic ataxia of Charlevoix–Saguenay (SACS) | Spasticity, severe neuropathy, no common association with movement disorders | <10 Late-onset possible |
| Ataxia telangiectasia (ATM) | Oculomotor apraxia, conjunctival telangiectasias, extrapyramidal signs, predisposition to cancer. Variable hyperkinesias, mainly dystonia, that may be levodopa-responsive | 2–3 Late-onset possible |
| Ataxia with oculomotor apraxia type 1 (APTX) | Like ataxia telangiectasia, sensorimotor neuropathy, chorea, cognitive impairment. Dystonia, chorea, parkinsonism | <20 Late-onset possible |
| Ataxia with oculomotor apraxia type 2 (SETX) | Like AOA1, some features to a lesser degree. Dystonia, chorea, parkinsonism | <20 Late-onset possible |
| Cerebrotendinous xanthomatosis (CYP27) | Pyramidal or extrapyramidal signs, seizures, dementia, juvenile cataract, tendon xanthomas. Parkinsonism, corticobasal syndrome, dystonia, myoclonus | <20 Late-onset possible |
| SANDO/MIRAS (POLG1) | Ophthalmoplegia, neuropathy, encephalopathy. Parkinsonism, myoclonus, dystonia | 15–40 |

# Fragile X-associated tremor/ataxia syndrome

### Fragile X syndrome
Fragile X syndrome is an inherited condition causing mental retardation. It is due to a triplet repeat expansion in the fragile site mental retardation (*FMR1*) gene on chromosome Xq27.3. Gene testing is available as a clinical service.

More than 200 repeats lead to loss of function of the *FMR1* gene and the development of mental retardation in affected males.

MRI of the brain usually shows a characteristic pattern of white matter hyperintensity in the middle cerebellar peduncles (MCP sign) and brainstem, as well as other, more non-specific, white matter lesions and generalized atrophy.

### Fragile X pre-mutation carriers
- Males with expansions of 55–200 repeats (fragile X pre-mutation carriers) can develop a movement disorder (usually tremor) and ataxia, with a typical age at onset of around 50 years—fragile X-associated tremor/ataxia syndrome (FXTAS).
- Female pre-mutation carriers have also been reported with FXTAS and are now recognized to occur more commonly than thought in the past. Premature ovarian failure is common in these women.
- Cognitive decline occurs in FXTAS but may not be severe.
- Tremor in FXTAS is usually an intention or action tremor.
- Postural and resting tremor has been reported in FXTAS, sometimes with no ataxia, leading to confusion with ET or PD.
- Other movement disorders have been reported with FXTAS, including dystonia and parkinsonism (which may be levodopa-responsive). Some patients have a combination of cerebellar signs, levodopa-unresponsive parkinsonism, and autonomic dysfunction, leading to diagnostic confusion with MSA.
- MRI may show similar abnormalities to those seen in full fragile X syndrome. This is more commonly seen in male pre-mutation carriers but is usually absent in female carriers.

# Other causes of movement disorder and ataxia

### Progressive ataxia palatal tremor syndrome
Some patients with palatal tremor (➲ p. 137) can also develop progressive ataxia. This PAPT is clinically heterogeneous and is due to a variety of causes.

Familial cases have been reported, usually with dominant inheritance. Such patients often have marked brainstem and cervical cord atrophy and pyramidal signs. Some will also have calcification or iron deposition in the dentate nucleus, leading to the use of the term 'dark dentate disease' to describe them. Rare families with PAPT have been reported due to Alexander disease, with mutations in the glial fibrillary acidic protein (*GFAP*) gene. Sporadic cases of PAPT have been reported secondary to lesions affecting the structures in and around the Guillain–Mollaret triangle (➲ p. 137).

### Coeliac disease
*Coeliac disease* has been associated with a progressive cerebellar syndrome, with or without movement disorders, such as cortical myoclonus and chorea, and dementia. Coeliac-associated neurological disorders are a controversial entity, as autoantibodies associated with coeliac disease are common in the asymptomatic general population, and some authors propose that coeliac-associated ataxia and movement disorders may occur by chance. The gold standard of diagnosis of coeliac disease is small bowel biopsy, and some have reported a response of the ataxia and movement disorders to a gluten-free diet.

### Glucose transporter 1 deficiency
GLUT1 deficiency has been covered in Chapter 11. Notably, apart from the typical phenotype, GLUT1 may present with a progressive ataxia spasticity syndrome that may also include dystonia, tremor, and cognitive decline. This syndrome may be treatable with a ketogenic diet.

## Useful websites and addresses

- **Ataxia UK**: Lincoln House, Kennington Park, 1–3 Brixton Road, London SW9 6DE. Tel: 0207 582 1444; http://www.ataxia.org.uk.
- **European Federation of Hereditary Ataxias**: http://www.euro-ataxia.eu.
- **National Ataxia Foundation (USA)**: http://www.ataxia.org.
- **Neuromuscular Disease Center (USA)**: http://neuromuscular.wustl.edu/. Website provided by the Washington University Neuromuscular Department; gives an excellent overview of ataxia in general, and is particularly helpful for summarizing the current state of genetic knowledge in this complex area.
- **EUROSCA**: http://www.eurosca.org.
- **International Parkinson and Movement Disorder Society**: http://www.movementdisorders.org.

# Chapter 13

# Movement disorders and sleep

Introduction *292*
Restless legs syndrome and periodic limb
 movements of sleep *294*
REM-sleep behaviour disorder *298*
Other conditions *300*
Useful websites and addresses *302*

## Introduction

Most movement disorders, with the exception of myoclonus and hemifacial spasm, disappear or greatly attenuate during sleep. However, other abnormal movements can emerge during sleep, either as a primary phenomenon or in association with another underlying movement disorder such as PD. In addition, some movement disorders are associated with excessive daytime sleepiness or insomnia.

A history from the patient's bed partner is very helpful in the assessment of movement disorders during sleep. The patient themselves may not be aware of the problem and may simply report excessive daytime sleepiness because of poor quality of sleep. Movement disorders during sleep are often a very early symptom of another underlying movement disorder, such as PD or MSA, but may be overlooked, unless specific enquiry is made during history taking.

Table 13.1 lists the causes of movement disorders which occur during sleep, and movement disorders which may be associated with sleep disturbance.

**Table 13.1** Movement disorders and sleep

| Disorder | Causes |
| --- | --- |
| Periodic limb movements of sleep (often associated with restless legs syndrome) | Idiopathic<br>Parkinson's disease<br>Low ferritin<br>Neuropathy<br>Hyperthyroidism |
| REM-sleep behaviour disorder | Parkinson's disease<br>Multiple system atrophy<br>Progressive supranuclear palsy<br>Dementia with Lewy bodies |
| Myoclonus | Hypnic jerks<br>Benign neonatal sleep myoclonus<br>*Jactatio capitis nocturnis*<br>Myoclonus that occurs during waking hours from any cause can also persist in sleep |
| Dystonia | Frontal lobe seizures<br>Autosomal dominant nocturnal frontal lobe epilepsy<br>'Off period' dystonia in Parkinson's disease |
| Excessive daytime somnolence | Parkinson's disease<br>Dementia with Lewy bodies<br>Treatment with dopamine agonists or levodopa<br>Periodic limb movements of sleep<br>REM-sleep behaviour disorder<br>Narcolepsy with cataplexy |
| Insomnia | Dementia with Lewy bodies (sleep inversion)<br>Encephalitis lethargica (sleep inversion)<br>Treatment with amantidine<br>Treatment with selegiline<br>Familial fatal insomnia |

# Restless legs syndrome and periodic limb movements of sleep

RLS and PLMS are common overlapping conditions, characterized by an urge to move the legs occurring during the evening (RLS) or abnormal movements of the legs during non-REM sleep (PLMS). RLS is also known as Ekbom's syndrome.

### Restless legs syndrome

*Clinical features*
- A common disorder, with mild symptoms affecting up to 11% of the population and clinically significant symptoms affecting about 3.5%.
- Typically, patients with RLS complain of unpleasant sensations in the legs occurring when at rest in the evening, made worse by fatigue or alcohol and relieved by limb movement. For example, patients can find it impossible to sit still to watch television in the evening or may have difficulty getting to sleep due to the constant need to move their legs.

*Diagnostic features of restless legs syndrome*
- An urge to move the legs, usually accompanied by unpleasant sensation in the legs.
- Symptoms occur during rest.
- Symptoms are relieved by moving the legs.
- Symptoms are worse in the evening or at night.

*Causes*
- RLS can occur as a primary phenomenon, usually with an autosomal dominant inheritance and teenage onset; however, no single monogenic cause has been identified. Genome-wide association studies identified six genetic variants, including MEIS1 and BTBD9, with potential relationships with iron metabolism.
- Secondary causes include pregnancy, iron deficiency anaemia, peripheral neuropathy (e.g. in patients with renal failure, diabetes), PD, hyperthyroidism, and multiple sclerosis. A variety of drugs may cause secondary RLS such as interferon alpha, levothyroxine, neuroleptics, or tricyclic antidepressants

*Pathophysiology*
- Pathological studies suggest defective iron metabolism and low iron levels in neuronal cells, particularly in the substantia nigra. Dysregulation of iron uptake and storage within brain microvessels has been reported recently and might play a role in a subgroup of RLS patients. Magnetic resonance studies using iron-sensitive sequences have demonstrated reduced iron content in several regions of the brain of RLS patients.
- Dopaminergic dysfunction has also been suggested as a cause of RLS, given the response of many RLS patients to dopaminergic drugs. Neuropathological studies have shown significant decreases in dopamine D2 receptors in the putamen that correlated with RLS

severity, and increased tyrosine hydroxylase in the substantia nigra. An overly activated dopaminergic system was reported in both animal and cell models of iron insufficiency. PET and SPECT studies support a dysfunction of dopaminergic pathways, involving not only the nigrostriatal pathway, but also the mesolimbic pathway.
- Functional MRI studies have demonstrated a pathologic activation of cerebral areas belonging to both the sensorimotor and limbic networks. Proton magnetic resonance spectroscopy has confirmed abnormality of the limbic system.

### Investigation
- Routine investigation of patients with RLS should include serum ferritin and a clinical examination to exclude neuropathy. Patients should be examined for signs of parkinsonism.

### Treatment
- Dopaminergic drugs (levodopa, pramipexole, ropinirole, rotigotine) are suggested as first-line treatment for RLS.
- $\alpha 2\delta$ ligands (gabapentin, gabapentin enacarbil, and pregabalin) have been shown to be efficacious in several studies.
- 'Augmentation' or 'rebound' phenomena can occur where symptoms worsen and occur earlier in the day, 6–12 months after starting treatment. This has been reported mainly with levodopa treatment but also occurs with dopamine agonists. In contrast, $\alpha 2\delta$ ligands may show less augmentation than dopaminergic drugs, but this needs to be confirmed in larger studies.
- Treatment with iron in patients with low serum ferritin may improve symptoms. Iron supplementation in those with normal serum ferritin is not of proven benefit.
- Opioids and clonazepam are used for the treatment of severe RLS when other drugs have failed; however, evidence is not sufficient for their use. Prolonged-release oxycodone–naloxone has been shown to be efficacious for short-term treatment of patients with severe RLS inadequately controlled with previous treatment.

## Periodic limb movements of sleep
- This disorder often occurs with RLS but may occur alone.
- Patients experience jerky flexion movements of the hips, knees, and ankles during non-REM sleep.
- Patients will often not be aware of the movements but may report daytime somnolence due to the frequent partial wakenings caused by the limb movements.
- PLMS are different from the movements seen in RBD (➔ p. 298). In PLMS, the movements are simple repetitive flexion movements, rather than the complex movements seen in RBD, and patients do not shout out or engage in coordinated behaviour.
- Causes are as for RLS, and treatment is similar, although clonazepam is the first-line treatment for isolated PLMS.

### How to introduce medications commonly used for the treatment of restless legs syndrome and periodic limb movements of sleep

*Ropinirole*

- Available in 0.25 mg, 1 mg, 2 mg, and 5 mg tablets, or Adartrel® (this is the trade name for the formulation of ropinirole specifically marketed for RLS) in 0.25 mg, 0.5 mg, and 2 mg tablets.
- Starting dose is 0.25 mg taken in the evening 1–2 hours before the usual onset of symptoms.
- Dose can be increased by 0.25 mg every 4–5 days to reach 1.5–2.5 mg daily. Adartrel® is available in a 'starter pack' which takes the patient to 2 mg daily over 7 days.
- Average effective daily dose in clinical trials was 2 mg/day.
- Main side effects are nausea, sedation (including sleep attacks), confusion, peripheral oedema, hypotension, and hallucinations.

*Pramipexole*

- Available in 0.125 mg, 0.25 mg, 0.5 mg, and 1 mg tablets.
- Starting dose is 0.125 mg taken in the evening 1–2 hours before the usual onset of symptoms (see previous explanation of salt equivalents).
- Dose can be increased, if necessary, in 0.125 mg increments every 7 days to reach 0.5–1 mg daily (see previous explanation of salt equivalents).
- Average effective daily dose in clinical trials was 0.75 mg/day.
- Main side effects are nausea, sedation (including sleep attacks), confusion, peripheral oedema, hypotension, and hallucinations.

*Rotigotine*

- Available as patch in 1 mg, 2 mg, 3 mg, 4 mg, 6 mg, and 8 mg.
- Starting dose is 1 mg/24 hours and can be increased every 2 weeks by 1 mg. However, usually the dose should not exceed 4 mg/24 hours.
- Main side effects are similar to other dopamine agonists. In addition, a skin reaction from the patch may occur.

*Clonazepam*

- Available in 500 micrograms (beige) or 2 mg (white) tablets. Tablets scored twice.
- Starting dose is 250 micrograms once in the evening (125 micrograms in the elderly). For PLMS, the dose should be taken 30 minutes before bedtime.
- Increase every week by 250 micrograms to reach 500 micrograms to 2 mg in the evening.
- Main side effects are sedation, depression, and fatigue.

# REM-sleep behaviour disorder

## Clinical features
RBD is a parasomnia characterized by the absence of normal muscle tone loss during REM sleep. This results in individuals 'acting out' their dreams. Normally, atonia during REM sleep is produced by active inhibition of motor pathways by pontine structures.

The bed partners of those with RBD usually report unusual behaviour during sleep, which can include shouting out, apparently purposeful limb movement, and even violent behaviour. Patients may report finding themselves on the floor in the middle of the night, having thrown themselves out of bed. Patients often report very vivid dreams. Sleep tends to be poor in RBD, and therefore patients may report daytime somnolence and fatigue.

## Common causes of REM-sleep behaviour disorder
- Primary or idiopathic RBD.
- PD.
- DLB.
- MSA.

RBD may be the presenting feature of parkinsonian disorders, sometimes occurring some years, and up to decades, prior to the onset of other symptoms.

## REM-sleep behaviour disorder and neurodegeneration
- RBD has been associated with diverse neurodegenerative disorders, but the most prominent association exists with the alpha-synucleinopathies.
- In patients with RBD, the risk of developing neurodegeneration is approximately 25–40% at 5 years and 40–65% at 10 years.
- A patient with typical RBD has a 50% chance of developing a parkinsonian syndrome within 5 years, most likely PD.
- Forty per cent of patients with PD, and 80–95% of patients with MSA, will have RBD.
- Patients with RBD have been found to have a higher prevalence of autonomic dysfunction, depression, mild cognitive changes, and olfactory loss than healthy controls.
- Patients with RBD may have abnormal dopamine transporter imaging, hyperechogenicity of the substantia nigra on ultrasound, and functional MRI studies similar to early-stage PD.
- Thus, at least a subset of patients with idiopathic RBD can represent a prodromal stage of PD or other synucleinopathies.
- The speed and amplitude of movements during RBD in patients with PD and MSA is often better than their movements when awake.

## Investigation and treatment

A typical history from the patient (and their partner), particularly in the context of a parkinsonian disorder, is usually sufficient to make the diagnosis. Polysomnography with video recording during sleep can be helpful in some cases, in particular for the differential diagnosis from other parasomnias. Treatment of the underlying parkinsonian condition can be helpful for RBD symptoms (e.g. dopaminergic drugs for PD). Clonazepam and melatonin are often helpful.

# Other conditions

## Seizures
Seizures, in particular frontal lobe seizures, can produce abnormal movement during sleep. Polysomnography can be helpful in the diagnosis of nocturnal seizures, although frontal lobe seizures can sometimes be difficult to detect with surface EEG. Dystonic spasms can occur at night (paroxysmal nocturnal dystonia), but these patients will almost all have frontal seizures as the cause. Such seizures can occur as a result of the familial syndrome of ADNFLE, which is discussed in Chapter 11 (➲ p. 273).

## Myoclonus
Myoclonus can persist during sleep, and therefore patients with daytime myoclonus may also have myoclonic jerks when asleep. Hypnic jerks (myoclonic jerks occurring on falling asleep or less commonly on waking) are a common normal phenomenon. Infants may have myoclonus during sleep (benign neonatal sleep myoclonus) which, as the name suggests, is benign and self-limiting. Some children have head-banging movements while falling asleep (*jactatio capitis nocturnis*), which is usually a benign and self-limiting phenomenon, commonly seen in the setting of mental retardation.

## Disruption of normal sleep patterns in association with movement disorders
Some movement disorder syndromes are associated with disruption of normal sleep patterns. Patients with DLB (➲ p. 36) and encephalitis lethargica (➲ p. 121) can experience periods of insomnia and reversal of the normal sleep–wake cycle, so that they are awake all night and sleep during the day. Patients with PD, particularly those with the 'dopamine dysregulation syndrome' where patients take very high doses of dopaminergic drugs, can experience insomnia. Both selegiline and amantadine can act as stimulants and therefore can disrupt sleep in patients with PD using these drugs.

Patients with PD often complain of daytime somnolence. This can be a consequence of poor sleep at night, due to PLMS, RBD, rigidity, or 'off-period' dystonia. However, it is often, in retrospect, the first harbinger of cognitive impairment, followed by hallucinations or complaints about memory. Some patients with PD can develop abnormal respiratory patterns similar to those seen in obstructive sleep apnoea, which can result in daytime somnolence. Dopamine agonists and levodopa are associated with hypersomnolence, and even 'sleep attacks' where patients will suddenly, and without warning, fall asleep during the day. Patients should be clearly warned and routinely asked about this side effect at clinic visits.

## Movement disorder in children with narcolepsy–cataplexy

Narcolepsy with cataplexy is characterized by daytime sleepiness, cataplexy (sudden loss of bilateral muscle tone triggered by emotions), sleep paralysis, hypnagogic hallucinations, and disturbed nocturnal sleep. Narcolepsy with cataplexy is most often associated with human leucocyte antigen-DQB1*0602 and is caused by the loss of hypocretin-producing neurons in the hypothalamus of likely autoimmune aetiology.

Patients with narcolepsy with cataplexy may display a complex array of 'negative' (hypotonia) and 'active' (ranging from perioral movements to dyskinetic–dystonic movements or stereotypies) motor disturbances. This complex movement disorder is seen at disease onset and may vanish later in the course of the disease.

## Movement disorder in NMDA antibody encephalitis

Anti-NMDA receptor encephalitis presents with initial symptoms similar to acute psychosis and subsequent development of seizures, decreased level of consciousness, autonomic instability, hypoventilation, and a characteristic movement disorder found in up to 89% of patients, which usually consists of complex bilateral antigravity stereotyped movements of the arms, with perioral and eye movements, and, less frequently, involvement of the legs. In some patients, the presence of antibodies is associated with teratomas of the ovaries, in which case a surgical removal is required. The condition can be fatal without treatment (immunomodulation, plasmapheresis, or corticosteroids), and this distinct movement disorder may assist in identifying the disease. It is hypothesized that the movements represent a dissociative state.

## Status dissociatus

State dissociations are the consequence of errors in the normal process of moving between wakefulness, REM, and non-REM sleep. In those, elements of one state persist or are recruited erroneously into another state. Status dissociatus results from a complete breakdown of state-determining boundaries. Several conditions have been reported to lead to this state, including fatal familial insomnia, Morvan's syndrome, and delirium tremens (alcohol withdrawal).

The rare condition familial fatal insomnia is an inherited prion disease. In the early stages of the disease, insomnia occurs, together with autonomic disturbance, ataxia, myoclonus, and pyramidal signs. Later in the disease, excessive sleepiness may replace the insomnia. Patients may have complex movements.

Morvan's syndrome, caused by antibodies against voltage-gated potassium channel-associated proteins, is characterized by neuromyotonia, severe sleep disturbance, and other features of limbic encephalitis

## CHAPTER 13 **Movement disorders and sleep**

## Useful websites and addresses
- RLS-UK, PO Box 61702, London SE9 9DD. Helpline: 01634 260483 (M&Th 9–11) http://www.rls-uk.org.
- Restless Legs Syndrome Foundation (USA): http://www.rls.org.
- International Parkinson and Movement Disorder Society: http://www.movementdisorders.org.

# Chapter 14

# Other dyskinetic syndromes

Introduction *304*
Hemifacial spasm *306*
Other dyskinetic syndromes *310*

# Introduction

There are some distinct hyperkinetic movement disorder syndromes which do not fit well into other sections and are instead described in the following text. With the exception of hemifacial spasm, the majority of these are rare, but a passing knowledge of them is desirable.

### Miscellaneous dyskinetic syndromes
- Hemifacial spasm
- Hemi-masticatory spasm (with or without facial hemiatrophy)
- Painful legs and moving toes
- Oculo-masticatory myorhythmia
- Belly dancer's dyskinesia
- The dancing larynx syndrome
- The neck–tongue syndrome
- Dyskinetic movements of the ear
- Facio-brachial dystonic seizures (associated with LGI1 voltage-gated potassium channel antibody encephalitis)
- Facial myokymia

# Hemifacial spasm

## Clinical features
- Hemifacial spasm is a common condition affecting approximately 7–14 per 100 000. It is probably commoner in Chinese or Korean patients and, in this population, may also have an earlier age at onset (see Video 14.1: Hemifacial spasm).
- It is a peripherally generated involuntary muscle spasm that affects muscles innervated by the facial nerve.
- Onset is usually in the fourth or fifth decade, and females are more often affected than males. Idiopathic hemifacial spasm is associated with hypertension.
- Patients usually describe involuntary muscle twitching affecting the muscles around the eye at onset, and later spreading to involve other muscles on the same side of the face. A characteristic feature is that these muscle spasms are synchronous. Spasm occurs spontaneously but can be induced by peripheral stimulation (such as touch, cold, or wind) or facial movement.
- Although hemifacial spasm is not a form of dystonia, patients are catered for by the dystonia patient associations (p. 248).

## Causes
- **Idiopathic hemifacial spasm**: thought to be caused by 'irritation' of the facial nerve at the root exit zone by an aberrant blood vessel.
- **Structural lesions in the region of the facial nerve root exit zone** in the pontocerebellar angle, e.g. tumours such as schwannoma (also hearing loss), demyelination, Bell's palsy.

## Investigation
- An MRI scan of the brain is the only investigation needed in clinically typical cases. In idiopathic hemifacial spasm, an ectatic tortuous blood vessel close to the facial nerve is sometimes seen.

## Treatment
*Botulinum toxin*
- BT injections into the affected muscles is the first-line treatment for hemifacial spasm. These give excellent results in 80–90% of patients, with few side effects.
- The effect of injections will wear off after 3–4 months and will need repeating to maintain the effect.
- Prior to injection, it should be explained that facial muscle weakness can be a long-term consequence of the hemifacial spasm itself. BT injections can cause a transient worsening of this weakness, but the underlying condition itself is responsible for any persistent weakness.
- The muscle anatomy of the face is given in Fig. 14.1, as a guide to injection placement.
- It is best to start by just giving injections to muscles around the eye. This may cause sufficient resolution of symptoms on its own. Treatment of muscle spasm around the mouth is difficult, as unacceptable facial weakness often results.

- Because they already have a partial irritative lesion of their facial nerve, patients with hemifacial spasm seem to be more sensitive to increases in BT dose than patients with dystonia, and therefore dose escalation should be performed with care.

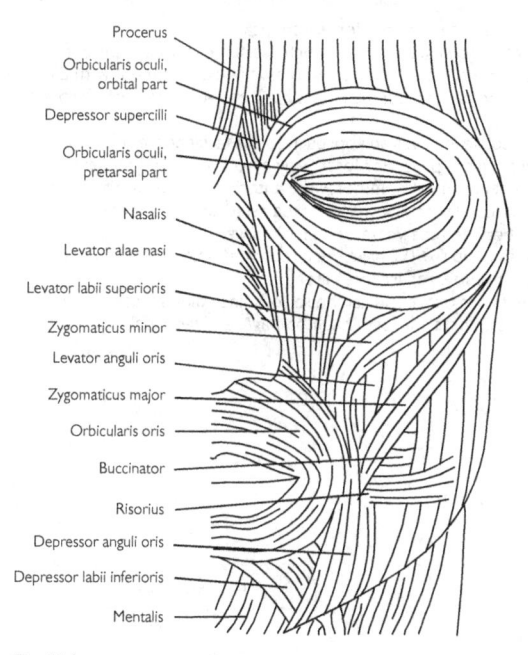

**Fig. 14.1** Muscle anatomy of the face as a guide for botulinum toxin injections in hemifacial spasm. In practice, injections into the orbicularis oculi, similar to those used in blepharospasm (Fig. 9.4), are sufficient for the vast majority of patients. Injection of other muscles of the face often leads to facial weakness, unless great care is taken with the dose selection and injection site.

*Medication*
- Prior to the introduction of BT, a variety of medications were used to treat hemifacial spasm, most often clonazepam and carbamazepine. In general, these had poor effectiveness and are now rarely used.

*Surgery*
- Posterior fossa decompression is a surgical approach to the treatment of hemifacial spasm, which has some limited application.
- It may be appropriate for those who have failed treatment with BT or those who wish to pursue a possible curative procedure, despite the risks.
- The procedure involves an approach to the facial nerve root exit zone through the posterior fossa. Any blood vessels adjacent to the facial nerve (most commonly the anterior inferior or posterior inferior cerebellar arteries) are moved aside, and a Teflon™ graft is inserted between the vessel and facial nerve.
- Cure rates of up to 90% have been reported (in retrospective case series), with a low recurrence rate.
- Side effects can occur and can be serious, including sensorineural hearing loss, posterior fossa haemorrhage, and facial palsy.

# Other dyskinetic syndromes

### Hemi-masticatory spasm
Hemi-masticatory spasm is characterized by bursts of involuntary muscle activity affecting the masseter on one side of the face. It is typically an idiopathic condition, thought to have an aetiology similar to hemifacial spasm, with irritation of the trigeminal motor nerve by an aberrant vessel. Some patients with hemi-masticatory spasm have been reported to have ipsilateral progressive facial hemiatrophy. Treatment with carbamazepine and BT has been reported to be effective.

### Painful legs and moving toes
- This (for once) clearly named condition is characterized by patients who complain of neuropathic pain (burning) in the legs and feet, accompanied by involuntary movements of the toes (see Video 14.2: Painful legs and moving toes).
- The movements are often quite small and writhing in nature, and can vary in amplitude. Usually pain precedes the onset of the abnormal movements. They are usually bilateral but can be unilateral. Repositioning of the affected limb can temporarily relieve the pain, but the abnormal movements usually continue unabated.
- A number of precipitating factors have been identified, including spinal cord, root, and plexus injury, peripheral neuropathy (in particular neuropathy associated with HIV infection), and soft tissue and bony injury. In other cases, no precipitating cause can be found.
- A syndrome of painful arms and moving fingers is also described, which is an analogous syndrome to painful legs and moving toes, but affecting the upper limbs.
- The major differential diagnosis is with focal myoclonus due to a cortical lesion (where pain is unlikely to be present and EEG may be abnormal) and spinal segmental myoclonus, or myoclonus secondary to root or plexus injury (where pain may be present). The characteristics of the abnormal movements are different in these myoclonic syndromes, and this can be demonstrated using EMG.
- Investigation should include imaging of the relevant part of the cord and plexus, and nerve conduction studies.
- Treatment of painful legs and moving toes is notoriously difficult. Numerous drugs, including antiepileptics (usually carbamazepine or gabapentin), benzodiazepines, and tricyclic antidepressants, have been tried, but with limited effect. Lumbar sympathetic blockade may be helpful. Spontaneous remission is rare.

### Other dyskinetic syndromes
- **Oculo-masticatory myorhythmia (OMM):** is a disorder characterized by synchronous 2 Hz vergence spasms of the eyes with contraction of the masseter. Palatal tremor may also be present. OMM is virtually pathognomonic of Whipple's disease.
- **Facio-brachial dystonic seizures:** are frequent, brief dystonic seizure-like movements affecting usually the arm and ipsilateral face,

associated with voltage-gated potassium channel (VGKC) complex/ LGI1 antibodies and, most importantly, commonly precede the onset of limbic encephalitis. Their recognition should prompt testing for these antibodies and treatment with immunotherapies, which may prevent the development of full-blown limbic encephalitis with its potential for cerebral atrophy and cognitive impairment.
- **Belly dancer's dyskinesia**: is a term coined in 1990 to describe patients with focal dyskinetic movements affecting muscles of the abdomen, leading to writhing movements of the abdominal wall. This condition may follow abdominal surgery or other abdominal trauma. There is one report of belly dancer's dyskinesia following the use of a DRB. Differential diagnoses include spinal and propriospinal myoclonus. Few data on treatment are available. Benzodiazepines, DRBs, BT, and stimulation of the abdomen with transcutaneous electrical stimulation (TENS) have been reported to be of help.
- **The neck–tongue syndrome**: is a rare condition, described by Orrell and Marsden in 1994. This syndrome is characterized by pseudo-athetoid movements of the tongue, pain in the neck exacerbated by movement, and paraesthesiae affecting the ipsilateral side of the tongue. The syndrome is thought to arise from damage to lingual afferent fibres travelling in the hypoglossal nerve via the C2 spinal roots. Most patients with the neck–tongue syndrome have evidence of pathology at the atlanto-axial or atlanto-occipital joints.
- **The dancing larynx syndrome** (non-rhythmic movements of the laryngeal cage in multiple directions): is rare and usually presents as part of a symptomatic palatal tremor–myoclonus syndrome.
- **Dyskinetic movements of the ear**: can be seen. These movements may be voluntary, occur as a tic, or occur as part of cranio-cervical dystonia.
- **Facial myokymia**: comprises involuntary activation of muscle fibres, with a characteristic EMG pattern. Facial myokymia is associated with brainstem lesions and can be seen, for example, in multiple sclerosis. Myokymia can be due to voltage-gated potassium channel antibodies (e.g. in Morvan's fibrillary chorea), EA1 (*KCNA1* mutations), or as part of a disorder called familial dyskinesia facial myokymia (FDFM), for which recently a causative gene has been identified (adenylyl cyclase 5, *ADCY5* mutations (→ p. 276)).

# Chapter 15

# Functional (psychogenic) movement disorders

Introduction and approach *314*
Features of functional movement disorders *316*
Functional tremor *318*
Functional dystonia *320*
Functional parkinsonism *322*
Functional myoclonus *324*
Management of functional movement disorders *326*
Useful websites *328*

# Introduction and approach

Functional disorders are common in neurological practice. Since the explosion of interest in functional disorders in the nineteenth century with Charcot and his followers, the diagnosis and treatment of functional disorders has been the subject of intense debate and controversy.

The diagnosis of functional movement disorders (FMDs) is often said to be difficult, and certainly there are patients where this is the case. However, there are many others where the application of a good general knowledge of movement disorders in general and an understanding of positive clinical signs in patients with FMDs makes the diagnostic process straightforward.

## Approach to patients with suspected functional movement disorders

There are common pitfalls in the approach to patients with suspected FMD. Many doctors have a view of FMD that is strongly influenced by a specific aetiological theory—that functional symptoms are caused by the conversion of psychological conflict into physical symptoms. This can lead the unwary clinician into making the diagnosis of FMD just because the patients is anxious/depressed/odd in personality or has suffered emotional trauma, and conversely failing to consider this diagnosis if the patient appears psychologically 'normal'. Diagnosis of FMD should not rest on the presence or absence of psychopathology. Another common pitfall is that doctors fail to make the diagnosis unless every other diagnostic possibility, however remote, has been excluded. This 'machine gun' approach to investigation can be directly harmful to a patient with FMD. Exhaustive (and often invasive) testing is time-consuming, carries risks, and tends to reinforce the idea in the mind of the patient that the condition must be organic. Testing of this sort will often throw up spurious abnormal results, which may be latched on to by the patient as further evidence of organicity of the condition. The time delay involved in this kind of approach also fails the patient by delaying the onset of appropriate treatment and generates considerable uncertainty.

A rational approach to FMD is to consider that this is a common cause of presentation to neurology clinics, especially specialist clinics, and, where at all possible, diagnosis should be based on the presence of positive features in the history and examination. This approach needs to be informed by a thorough knowledge and familiarity with the range of organic movement disorders and their presentation. This provides a firm base from which to identify patients with symptoms and signs that do not fit recognized patterns of organic movement disorders, and therefore where a functional disorder needs to be considered in the differential diagnosis. Targeted and limited investigations often have a place in the assessment of these patients, and this process can, in many cases, lead to sufficient diagnostic certainty.

## Elliot Slater and long-term follow-up of functional illness

In 1965, Elliot Slater published two influential papers regarding 10 years of follow-up on patients diagnosed with functional neurological symptoms.[1,2] Fifty per cent of patients were said to have developed clear-cut psychiatric or organic neurological conditions during follow-up. This study encouraged the reluctance of many clinicians to diagnose functional illness for fear of missing an underlying organic diagnosis.

However, the issue was revisited in 1998 in a 6-year follow-up of 73 patients diagnosed with functional neurological symptoms, with face-to-face interviews and analysis of GP and hospital records conducted to determine if an organic diagnosis had been made that explained the original symptoms. Only three cases were found to have organic diagnoses that explained their original symptoms at follow-up.[3]

1 Slater E (1965). Diagnosis of 'hysteria'. *BMJ*, i, 1395–9.

2 Slater ET, Glithero E (1965). A follow-up of patients diagnosed as suffering from 'hysteria'. *J Psychosom Res*, 9, 9–13.

3 Crimlisk HL, Bhatia K, Cope H, David A, Marsden CD, Ron MA (1998). Slater revisited: 6 year follow up study of patients with medically unexplained motor symptoms. *BMJ*, 316, 582–6.

# Features of functional movement disorders

## Epidemiology of functional movement disorders
Functional illness is a common cause of movement disorders. In general neurology clinics, FMDs account for up to 2% of all patients, whereas, in tertiary specialist movement disorder clinics, FMDs may account for over 20% of patients. Women are more likely to develop FMDs than men (2–4:1). Typical age at onset is in young adults (twenties and thirties) but varies widely. FMDs are less common, but still occur, in the young (<10 years) and the elderly (>70 years).

## Types of functional movement disorders
The proportion of patients with different FMDs is variable. The commonest are functional tremor and dystonia, followed by functional myoclonus and parkinsonism. Functional chorea and tics are very rare. Functional paroxysmal movement disorders have also been described and overlap with patients with non-epileptic seizures.

## Clinical features suggestive of a functional movement disorder
Clinical criteria for confidence in diagnosing an FMD have been proposed and are given in Box 15.1. There are a number of features in the history and examination which provide support for the diagnosis of FMD, regardless of the particular movement disorder seen.

### History
- Sudden onset of symptoms, with rapid progression to maximum
- Waxing and waning of symptoms, with sudden remissions and reappearances of symptoms, often in different body parts
- Paroxysmal exacerbations of symptoms and shift in phenomenology over time
- Multiple additional neurological and systemic symptoms
- Presence of an identifiable physical or psychological precipitating event to the emergence of symptoms or worsening of symptoms

### Examination
- Resolution or diminution of symptoms with distraction
- Exacerbation of symptoms when the affected body part is examined
- Improvement of symptoms with suggestion
- 'Give-way' weakness of the limbs
- Functional patterns of sensory disturbance
- Functional patterns of speech disturbance
- Excessive response to startle
- Disability out of proportion to examination findings
- Functional gait disturbance

## Gait disturbance in functional movement disorders

Gait disturbance is a common accompaniment to FMDs. It is often a useful clinical feature that discriminates between functional and organic movement disorders, and a thorough assessment of gait is essential. A variety of gait problems are seen, alone or in combination, including the following.

- **Astasia/abasia (also known as 'tightrope walker gait' or 'walking on ice gait')**: here, the patient dramatically veers from side to side when walking, often waving the arms at the same time. Patients continually seem to be about to lose their balance but tend not to do so. In fact, such gait demonstrates very good balance, as the patient is able to shift their centre of gravity quickly from side to side without falling.
- **Narrow base**: in contrast to many other patients with poor balance, patients with functional gait disturbance tend to walk with a narrow, rather than a broad, base.
- Hesitation.
- Dramatic response to Romberg's test and tests of postural stability.
- Excessive slowness.

---

**Box 15.1 Diagnostic criteria for the diagnosis of functional movement disorders**

*Documented*

Persistent relief by psychotherapy, suggestion, or placebo has been demonstrated, which may be helped by physiotherapy, or the patient was seen without the movement disorder when believing himself or herself unobserved.

*Clinically established*

The movement disorder is incongruent with a classical movement disorder, or it is inconsistent over time, plus at least one of the following: other functional signs, multiple somatizations, or an obvious psychiatric disturbance.

*Probable*

The movement disorder is inconsistent over time or incongruent with a typical movement disorder, or there are functional signs or multiple somatizations.

*Possible*

Evidence of an emotional disturbance.

Reproduced from *Neurology*, 65, Williams DT et al., Phenomenology and psychopathology related to functional movement disorders, pp. 231–257, Copyright (1995), with permission from Wolters Kluwer Health.

## Functional tremor

### Clinical features of functional tremor
Patients with functional tremor usually have clinical features common to all FMDs (📽 see Video 15.1: 'Psychogenic tremor'). Additional features of functional tremor are:
- often present at rest, on posture, and during action
- variable amplitude and frequency
- distractibility with rhythmic movements of the limbs
- it may entrain (match the frequency of) rhythmic movements of the limbs
- worsening when the limb is examined.

### Useful bedside tests for functional tremor
- **Distractibility and entrainment**: the key here is to ask the patient to match a rhythmic movement with their hand or foot at a pace which is set by the examiner. This 'externally paced' movement should cause a functional tremor to pause or change frequency. In entrainment, the tremor frequency shifts to match exactly that of the externally paced movement. Some patients will be unable to perform the simple tapping movement; this suggests an inability to shift attention away from the tremor and is another positive clinical sign. Head tremors are better distracted by rotatory movements of the arms or side-to-side movements of the tongue.
- **Pause with ballistic movement**: ask the patient to reach to your finger as quickly as possible when it is presented. This ballistic movement should produce a short pause in a functional tremor.
- **Loading**: the majority of organic tremors improve with loading of the affected limb. If patients with functional tremor of the arm are given weights to hold, their tremor usually worsens.
- **Restraint**: in patients with functional tremor, if the shaking limb is deliberately restrained by the examiner, the tremor tends to worsen and spread to other parts of the body.

### Useful investigations in functional tremor
- EMG of the tremor can be very helpful. This simple test provides objective evidence of variability of tremor frequency and response of the tremor to entrainment manoeuvres and loading.
- The differential diagnosis in some patients with functional tremor is PD. In such cases where there is diagnostic uncertainty, a DAT scan can be helpful. This will be normal in functional tremor but is abnormal in PD (and some other parkinsonian conditions). Remember, however, that DAT scans are normal in a number of organic conditions which cause tremor, including dystonia, ET, and tremor due to drugs.

## Functional dystonia

Functional dystonia is a common FMD. It is one of the most difficult FMDs to diagnose, as organic dystonia is an unusual condition itself, and there is still considerable controversy about whether certain types of dystonia are organic or functional.

### Clinical features of functional dystonia

Patients with functional dystonia usually have clinical features common to all FMDs (➔ p. 317) and may fulfil criteria for psychiatric disorders such as somatization disorder, conversion disorder, anxiety, and depression (📽 see Video 15.2: Fixed dystonic posture). Additional features of functional dystonia are:
- often a precipitating factor, e.g. minor trauma
- unusual distribution of dystonia, given the age at onset (e.g. generalized dystonia in an adult; ➔ p. 201)
- fixed postures, rather than the typical mobile postures of organic dystonia
- severe pain
- absence of task/position specificity
- absence of sensory geste
- poor response to BT.

### Useful bedside tests for functional dystonia

- **Distractibility**: ask the patient to close their eyes and perform a cognitive task (e.g. serial subtraction of 7 from 100, with the answers said aloud) or a repetitive movement task with a pace set by an external cue. This may reduce the abnormal posturing of functional dystonia but tends to exacerbate organic dystonia.

### Pitfalls in the diagnosis of functional dystonia

*Organic dystonia is unusual*
- Task specificity: organic dystonia may only appear during the performance of a particular task. Dystonia of the legs can appear only during particular actions (e.g. walking forward may be difficult, but walking backwards or running may be easier).
- Jerky, position-sensitive tremor: organic dystonic tremor tends to be jerky and of variable amplitude, and only occurs in particular positions of the limb.
- Sensory tricks: patients with organic dystonia can often relieve dystonic spasms to some extent by gently touching the affected body part.
- Response to stress: many patients with organic dystonia find that their symptoms are worse when they are stressed or anxious.

*Post-traumatic dystonia, causalgia–dystonia, and fixed dystonia*
- In post-traumatic dystonia, dystonic posturing of a limb occurs secondary to minor trauma. Dystonia may spread outside the affected area.
- Causalgia–dystonia is a condition where minor trauma causes dystonic posturing of the limb, together with severe pain and trophic changes in the limb (loss of hair, muscle wasting, skin colour changes).
- Both these phenomena are now commonly called 'fixed dystonia' due to the very common occurrence of fixed abnormal postures of the limbs (most often hands and feet), in contrast to the mobile abnormal postures seen in typical dystonia. Fixed postures are very unusual in typical dystonia outside the setting of structural lesions of the basal ganglia and neurodegenerative disease, e.g. CBD.
- Current consensus is that the majority of patients with post-traumatic fixed dystonia and causalgia–dystonia have a functional basis for their disorder. Such patients should be carefully assessed for supporting evidence for the diagnosis of an FMD. There is a common overlap with complex regional pain syndrome type 1. Benign joint hypermobility (Ehlers–Danlos syndrome type 3) appears to be a possible risk factor for the development of fixed dystonia.

# Functional parkinsonism

### Clinical features of functional parkinsonism
Patients with functional parkinsonism usually have clinical features common to all FMDs (➔ p. 317). Additional features of functional parkinsonism are as follows.
- Tremor is often a prominent feature and has features typical of other functional tremors (➔ p. 318).
- 'Rigidity' has the characteristics of voluntary stiffness, and the resistance often changes, depending on how fast the limb is moved.
- Although movements may be slow, the progressive fatiguing of movement seen with organic akinesia is usually absent. Movements are often extremely slow when the patient is being examined, but less so when they are distracted.
- Symptoms are usually symmetrical.
- Gait is often bizarre, with slowness and unsteadiness combined. Reduction in arm swing may occur, but usually because the arms are held tightly at the sides.
- Testing of postural stability often leads to dramatic loss of balance and falls.

### Useful bedside tests for functional parkinsonism
- **Tremor tests**: most patients with functional parkinsonism will have tremor, and this can be assessed as outlined (➔ p. 318).
- **Distractibility**: ask the patient to close their eyes and perform a cognitive task (e.g. serial subtraction of 7 from 100, with the answers said aloud). This tends to reduce rigidity in functional parkinsonism but increases rigidity in organic parkinsonism. Distractibility of tremor may be less useful, as functional overlay may be present.

### Useful investigations in functional parkinsonism
- A DAT scan can be useful where there is diagnostic uncertainty. This is abnormal in PD (and some other parkinsonian conditions) but will be normal in functional parkinsonism. However, note that DAT scans are normal in some organic parkinsonian conditions (e.g. drug-induced parkinsonism and DRD).

# Functional myoclonus

### Clinical features of functional myoclonus
Patients with functional myoclonus usually have clinical features common to all FMDs (→ p. 317). Additional features of functional myoclonus are:
- dramatic stimulus sensitivity of jerks (although stimulus sensitivity can be seen in organic myoclonus)
- variability in the distribution of jerks from day to day.

### Useful bedside tests for functional myoclonus
- **Distractibility/entrainability**: sometimes functional myoclonus occurs in a semi-rhythmic pattern. If the patient is asked to set up a rhythmic tapping with an unaffected limb, the pattern of the jerking can entrain to this, or break down and stop temporarily.

### Useful investigations in functional myoclonus
- **EMG**: organic myoclonic jerks are typically caused by very brief (<50 ms) bursts of muscle activity (although brainstem myoclonus can be of longer duration). It is not possible to consistently voluntarily produce an EMG burst of less than about 50–75 ms, and therefore a finding of bursts shorter than this supports the diagnosis of organic myoclonus.
- **Pre-movement EEG potentials**: prior to normal voluntary movement, a slow-rising wave called the *bereitschafts potential* (BP) is seen on the EEG. This can be looked for by performing an EEG during EMG recording of a number of jerks. The EEG trace shortly before each jerk is then selected and averaged, and this may reveal the presence of a BP in functional myoclonus.

# Management of functional movement disorders

### Explaining the diagnosis
- It is not sufficient for the clinician to reach the diagnosis of an FMD and then fail to communicate this to the patient.
- However, FMDs can be treatable, and, in those who fail to improve, a clear diagnosis greatly assists the process of long-term management.
- An explanation of the diagnosis is a treatment in its own right. One approach is as follows.
  - A clear statement of the diagnosis: 'You have a functional tremor…'
  - A statement that provides confidence in this diagnosis: 'This is a common cause of movement disorder. I see this very commonly.'
  - A statement that the symptoms are real and are not imagined or 'put on'.
  - A clear explanation of how the diagnosis was reached—this can be very much helped by demonstration of positive physical signs, e.g. the cessation of tremor with distraction.
  - An explanation of how the nature of functional symptoms (that they are a 'software', and not a 'hardware', problem) means that they have the theoretical capacity to improve.
  - An exploration of the possible triggering factors, e.g. physical illness/injury and psychological stress or difficulty. This needs to be approached with sensitivity.

### Treatment plans
Despite the high prevalence of FMDs, very little evidence exists regarding the best choice of treatment. Most treatment programmes rely on a combination of the following.

- **Physiotherapy**: this can be an effective treatment for patients with FMD. The approach is based on finding ways to trigger normal movement/more control over movement. Often the 'tricks' that are used to reduce symptoms as part of the diagnostic assessment (e.g. distractibility of functional tremor) can be adapted to help the patient gain more control of movement.
- **Psychiatric/psychological input**: assessment and treatment of underlying psychiatric disorders, where present, can be important. Cognitive behavioural therapy can be very effective, as can medical treatment of anxiety and depression, if present.
- **Demedicalization**: patients with FMD may be receiving treatment with numerous medications by the time they are diagnosed. A graded plan of medication withdrawal is important and may improve any drug-induced symptoms.
- **Management of pain and fatigue**: pain and fatigue are common counterparts of FMDs and, in some patients, can be the dominant problem. Such patients are best managed in close collaboration with specialist pain management services and fatigue services.

*Inpatient treatment*

Admission to hospital can be helpful for some patients with severe symptoms. Typically, patients develop a series of goals with therapists (physiotherapy, occupational therapy, and cognitive behavioural/psychological therapy), and an individualized plan is drawn up to help achieve these goals over an extended inpatient admission.

*Containment and long-term management*

There are a proportion of patients who do not improve, despite their, and their treating team's, best efforts. It is important for patients and their treating teams to realize that not all patients will get better with treatment. As with neurorehabilitation in general, knowing when to stop active treatment is as important as knowing when to start it. Such patients often benefit from intermittent contact with a neurologist and should be supported in the community with appropriate aids and input according to their disability.

There are some other patients who are entirely unwilling to accept a functional diagnosis for their symptoms. In such cases, the clinician has a very important role: to give a clear explanation of the diagnosis to the patient, the primary care physician, and any other therapists and doctors involved in the patient's care. This serves the very important purpose of containment, therefore helping to prevent further referrals to other doctors and therapists. Such consultations often result in further (invasive) tests, medical treatment, and perhaps even surgical procedures. Patients with functional illness are particularly vulnerable to unscrupulous medical practitioners and 'therapists', who may offer unnecessary investigations and treatment, often for financial gain.

## Prognostic factors in functional movement disorders

Poor prognostic factors for recovery from FMDs are:
- somatization disorder
- longer duration of symptoms
- loss of employment
- ongoing litigation
- poor social support.

## Useful websites
- Functional and dissociative neurological symptoms: a patient guide (UK): http://www.neurosymptoms.org.
- FND Hope (USA): http://www.fndhope.org.

# Chapter 16

# Startle and stiff-person syndromes

Startle syndromes *330*
Stiff-person syndromes: 1 *332*
Stiff-person syndromes: 2 *334*

# Startle syndromes

Startle is a normal brainstem reflex. One way of thinking about startle is that it is a reflex that places the body in a 'defensive posture', ready to deal with the potential threat from the unexpected stimulus. Following a stimulus that produces startle (e.g. a sudden loud noise), muscle activity starts in the sternomastoid and spreads up to the face and down to the arms and legs. This muscle activation occurs very quickly after the stimulus (40–50 ms). The normal startle response will quickly habituate. There are a number of neurological conditions where excessive startle occurs.

## Hyperekplexia

- Hyperekplexia is a dominantly inherited startle syndrome due to a mutation in the gene encoding the A1 subunit of the glycine receptor.
- Patients experience a 'hung-up jerk' when startled. This is a generalized myoclonic jerk followed by stiffening of the limbs. Patients will often fall, if standing.
- The startle response does not habituate.
- In some patients, this disabling condition can be treated effectively with clonazepam and sodium valproate.
- Antibodies against the A1 subunit of the glycine receptor have been identified as causative in patients with PERM who also present with hyperekplexia.

## Other startle syndromes

- Excessive startle can be seen following brainstem injury, most commonly if the injury involves the pons.
- Excessive startle is also seen in patients who are simply anxious and can rarely be a functional/psychogenic phenomenon. In this situation, the early startle response occurring before 75–100 ms after the stimulus is normal, but the late response happening after this time is abnormally large.
- Startle epilepsy is a condition in which patients have a normal startle response, but the startle will trigger a generalized epileptic seizure.
- The automatic obedience syndromes are rare conditions which have startle as their main feature. There is considerable debate as to whether such syndromes are neurological, psychiatric, or perhaps simply cultural. There are some suggestions that these syndromes may be an unusual presentation of TS (➔ p. 148).

The original description was by Beard in 1878 amongst lumberjacks of French Canadian descent working in Maine. These 'jumping Frenchmen of Maine' appeared to have had an exaggerated startle response. Following a startle response, they would tend to repeat any word said to them (echolalia) and to obey any command given to them. The syndrome appeared to run in families. Similar syndromes have been described in Malaysia (Latah) and Siberia (Myriachit).

# Stiff-person syndromes: 1

Stiffness, usually superimposed with violent spasms and exaggerated startle (hyperekplexia), is the hallmark features of stiff-person syndromes, which comprises a continuum from the stiff-limb syndrome to PERM.

## Stiff-person syndrome

### Historical aspects
The term 'stiff man syndrome' was coined by Moersch and Woltman in 1956, who described patients with fluctuating and progressive rigidity and painful muscle spasm leading to gait difficulties, falls, and a 'wooden man' appearance. In 1991, Jankovic changed the term to 'stiff-person syndrome' (SPS), as the syndrome could also occur in women. Subsequent studies established SPS as an autoimmune disorder most frequently associated with antibodies against GAD.

### Epidemiology
- SPS has an estimated prevalence of 1–2/1 000 000.
- Age at onset is usually between 20 and 50 years.
- Classical SPS affects women 2–3 times more often than men.

### Pathophysiology
- A dysfunction of gamma-aminobutyric acid (GABA), thus of inhibitory mechanisms, has been proposed to be caused by anti-GAD antibodies.
- GAD is the rate-limiting step in the decarboxylation of L-glutamate to GABA, and the inhibitory effect of anti-GAD antibodies on GABA synthesis has been confirmed experimentally.
- The pathogenic role of anti-GAD antibodies is disputed, because serum and CSF titres do not always correlate with clinical fluctuations and severity of SPS.
- Other antibodies are described. Antibodies against the $GABA_A$ receptor-associated protein are detected in up to 70% of patients with non-paraneoplasic SPS. This interacts with gephryin.
- Antiglycine receptor (GlyR) antibodies, most commonly associated with PERM (➔ p. 334), can be found in 10–15% of patients with SPS. Anti-amphiphysin antibodies have been found in patients with paraneoplastic SPS (➔ p. 334), particularly associated with breast cancer.

### Clinical picture of classic stiff-person syndrome
- Onset is usually insidious, with intermittent muscle tightness or pain affecting the trunk. Patients then develop stiffness, slow voluntary movements, muscle hypertrophy, and abnormal postures with a characteristic lumbar hyperlordosis.
- The stiffness progresses from the trunk to proximal, and then distal, limb muscles. Gait and balance problems with frequent falls can occur.
- Dyspnoea and early satiety can occur.

- Muscle spasms triggered by emotional stress, startle, or sudden movements.
- Depression, anxiety, and situation-specific phobias have been reported in around half of the cases.
- SPS patients may develop severe life-threatening complications, particularly if untreated, including paroxysmal autonomic dysfunction (high blood pressure, tachycardia, hyperthermia).

*Examination*
- There is a characteristic hyperlordosis with hypertrophy of the lumbar paraspinal muscles in many patients.
- Patients are classically unable to bend down and touch their toes.
- Generalized hyperreflexia, clonus, and upgoing plantar responses are seen.
- Muscle weakness and sensory signs are not part of classic SPS.
- Oculomotor dysfunction may be present (dysconjugate gaze, horizontal and vertical supranuclear gaze palsy, hypometric and slow saccades, impaired smooth pursuit, nystagmus, and abduction deficits).
- Exaggerated startle responses occur, with abnormal exteroceptive reflexes and disinhibition of brainstem reflexes (e.g. head retraction reflex).

*Investigation*
- EMG of affected muscles (typically the paraspinal muscles) shows 'continuous motor unit activity'. Remember that this can occur with continuous voluntary contraction of the muscles.

*Associated conditions*
- Patients with type 1 diabetes mellitus, Batten disease, autoimmune polyendocrine syndrome type 1, cerebellar ataxia, drug-refractory epilepsy, and palatal myoclonus can also have anti-GAD antibodies.
- Type 1 diabetes is observed in 30% of patients with SPS.
- In patients with SPS, anti-GAD antibodies are found in blood and the CSF, while these antibodies are only seen in blood of type 1 diabetes patients.

*Treatment*
Treatment is aimed at symptom relief and/or modulation of the underlying immune process. There remains an important role for a multidisciplinary approach to management, including physiotherapy and occupational therapy input.
- Symptomatic treatment includes benzodiazepines, baclofen, and dantrolene.
- IVIG or plasma exchange are the main strategies for immunomodulation.
- Corticosteroids, rituximab, and cyclophosphamide have been used, but formal studies are lacking.

# Stiff-person syndromes: 2

## Paraneoplastic stiff-person syndrome
- Neuropathy and encephalopathy are the commonest neurological manifestations in patients with anti-amphiphysin antibodies, but an SPS phenotype can also occur.
- These patients often have a rostro-caudal distribution of stiffness, with more frequent neck and upper limb stiffness, in contrast to classic non-paraneoplastic SPS.
- Rhabdomyolysis in patients with antibodies recognizing the brain and muscle isoforms of amphiphysin is a potential complication.
- Paraneoplastic SPS has been associated also with anti-GAD and anti-Ri (ANNA-2) antibodies. The underlying neoplasia is most commonly the breast, colon, lung, thymus, and non-Hodgkin's lymphoma.
- In paraneoplastic SPS, the underlying tumour should be looked for and treated.

## Stiff-limb syndrome
- In some cases, the syndrome is confined to one limb, more commonly the leg, which can, however, subsequently spread.
- Up to half of these patients have sphincter disturbance, and about a third develop brainstem involvement.
- Anti-GAD antibodies are found in most of these cases.
- Partial response to GABA-ergic treatment.
- Electrophysiological findings are similar to those in classical SPS.

## Progressive encephalomyelitis with rigidity and myoclonus

### Historical aspects
PERM was first described by Campbell and Garland in 1956 in three patients exhibiting axial and limb rigidity, with prominent myoclonus, accompanied by profuse sweating and hyperthermia.

### Clinical features
- Most patients present in the fifth or sixth decade of life with insidious onset and a relapsing–remitting course.
- Patients present with similar, but generally more severe, stiffness, as seen in SPS, accompanied by stimulus-sensitive myoclonus, ataxia and dysautonomia, e.g. sweating, tachycardia, and urinary retention. Some may have breathing and swallowing difficulties and psychiatric features.
- Antiglycine alpha-1 receptor (anti-GlyR) antibodies are typically found, although some patients also have anti-GAD antibodies.
- DPPX (dipeptidyl peptidase-like protein 6) antibodies have been identified recently as a new cause of PERM.
- An associated tumour is documented in about 20% of cases.
- The prognosis is variable. One-quarter of patients require mechanical ventilation, and mortality can be as high as 40%.
- Some cases show substantial and sustained improvement with immunotherapies, usually with combinations of corticosteroids, IVIG, plasma exchange, and cyclophosphamide.

# Index

## A

abetalipoproteinaemia 171, 284
acanthocytosis 170–1
aceruloplasminaemia 226–7
acetazolamide 274
acetylcholine 20
action myoclonus renal failure syndrome 187, 188
action tremor 124
acute dystonic reactions 230, 254, 255
ADHD 262
adult-onset isolated cranio-cervical dystonia 208–9, 235
adult-onset isolated limb dystonia 206, 234
adult-onset tourettism 148
akathisia 265
akinesia 22
akinetic crisis 264–5
akinetic–rigid syndrome, see parkinsonism
Alexander disease 288
alien-limb phenomena 108
alpha-synuclein 28, 42, 102, 114, 115
alpha-synucleinopathies 114
amantadine 64
amino acidaemias 219
*ANO3* 208
anterior cingulate loop 10
anti-basal ganglia antibodies (ABGAs) 121, 157
antibodies
 anti-basal ganglia (ABGAs) 121, 157
 anti-GAD 332
 anti-myelin-associated glycoprotein 130
 NMDA 173, 301
 voltage-gated potassium channel 301, 311
anticholinergics 64, 67
antidepressants 68
anti-GAD antibodies 332
anti-myelin-associated glycoprotein antibodies 130
anti-NMDA receptor encephalitis 173, 301
antiphospholipid syndrome 172
apathy 68

APO-go® PEN 82
apomorphine 59, 82–3
apraxia
 corticobasal degeneration 108
 eyelid opening 96, 242
aripiprazole 152, 153
astasia/abasia 317
astrocytes
 plaques 108
 tufted 96
ataxia 279–90
 abetalipoproteinaemia 284
 ataxia telangiectasia 218, 284
 autosomal recessive spastic ataxia of Charlevoix–Saguenay 284
 cerebellar 98, 215
 cerebrotendinous xanthomatosis 284
 coeliac disease 288
 dystonia 215, 219
 episodic 268, 276, 277
 fragile X-associated tremor/ataxia syndrome 286
 Friedreich's 283, 284
 GLUT1 deficiency 288
 hereditary with vitamin E deficiency 284
 inherited 282–4
 with oculomotor apraxia type 1/2 283, 284
 progressive ataxia palatal tremor syndrome 137, 288
 Refsum's disease 284
 SANDO/MIRAS 284
 spinocerebellar 219, 282
ataxia telangiectasia 218, 284
atherosclerosis 120
athetoid cerebral palsy 230
athetosis 160
*ATP1A3* 218
*ATP13A2* 44, 117, 226
atypical
 parkinsonism 93–122
 corticobasal degeneration 108–10, 112, 218
 degenerative causes 116–18
 multisystem atrophy 102–5, 112, 218

 progressive supranuclear palsy 96–9, 112, 218
 secondary parkinsonism 23, 94, 120–1
autism 156
autoimmune disease 161, 172–3
automatic activity 10
automatic obedience syndromes 330
autonomic symptoms 38, 69
autosomal dominant nocturnal frontal lobe epilepsy 273
autosomal recessive spastic ataxia of Charlevoix–Saguenay 284

## B

baclofen 236
ballism 160
Baltic myoclonus 186
basal ganglia
 calcification 116
 circuits 14–15
 lesions 35
 movement disorders 18
 neurotransmitters 20
 Parkinson's disease 18, 28
 structure and function 10
Batten's disease 186
Behçet's syndrome 173
belly dancer's dyskinesia 311
benign hereditary chorea 173
benign joint hypermobility 321
benign myoclonic epilepsy 184
benign neonatal sleep myoclonus 300
benign tremulous Parkinson's disease 73
benzhexol 64, 138, 236, 257
*bereitschafts* potential 181, 324
beta oscillations 18
beta-propeller protein-associated neurodegeneration 226

335

blepharospasm 209, 235, 242
botulinum toxin
 treatment 7
 drooling 69
 dystonia 238–42
 dystonic clenched fist 109
 hemifacial spasm 306
 Tourette's syndrome 152
 tremor 138
bouncy legs syndrome 176
Braak hypothesis 28
bradykinesia 22, 25
brain imaging, see imaging
brain injury/lesions
 chorea 161, 173
 dystonia 230
 parkinsonism 121
 tics 156
bromocriptine 59
Brueghel syndrome 208

## C

*C2orF37* 219
*C9ORF72* 117, 165
*CACNA1A* 276
camptocormia 22
carbamazepine 274
catechol-O-methyltransferase inhibitors 62
caudate 14, 150
causalgia–dystonia 321
cerebellar ataxia 98, 215
cerebellar syndromes 281
cerebellar tremor 134
cerebrospinal fluid analysis 210–11
cerebrotendinous xanthomatosis 284
ceruloplasmin levels 221
cervical dystonia 208, 235, 240
channelopathies 268
chin tremor 125, 137
chorea 2, 159–74
 acanthocytosis 170–1
 antiphospholipid syndrome 172
 autoimmune 161, 172–3
 benign hereditary 173
 brain lesions 161, 173
 causes 160, 161
 cerebellar syndrome 281
 definition 160
 drug-induced 161, 173, 258
 examination 162
 history-taking 162
 Huntington's disease 164–8
 investigation 162
 neuroacanthocytosis 170
 pregnancy 172
 senile 173
 Sydenham's 156, 172
 treatment 162
chorein 170
choreoathetosis 160
chronic inflammatory demyelinating polyradiculoneuropathy 130
chronic traumatic encephalopathy 121
*CIZ1* 208
clonazepam 139, 192, 236, 257, 296
clonidine 152, 153
clozapine 69, 256, 257
co-beneldopa 53
co-careldopa 53–4
cock walk 120
coeliac disease 165, 173, 191, 288
cogwheel rigidity 22
complex tics 142, 143
complex writer's cramp 206
computerized tomography (CT) 40
constraint-induced movement therapy 246
continuous dopaminergic stimulation 78
copper-chelating agents 222
copper levels 221
coprolalia 142
copropraxia 142
corticobasal degeneration 108–10, 112, 218
corticobasal syndrome 98, 109
Coxsackie B virus 121
cryptococcus 121
CSF analysis 210–11
*CSTB* 186
cycad plant 118

## D

dancing larynx syndrome 311
dantrolene sodium 264
dark dentate disease 288
DAT scan 40, 104, 109, 252, 318, 322
daytime somnolence 80, 293, 300
*DCTN1* 117
deafness 215, 219
deconditioning 66
deep brain stimulation 7
 dystonia 244

Parkinson's disease 86–7
Tourette's syndrome 153
tremor 138
degenerative disease
 chorea 161
 dystonia 214–16
 parkinsonism 116–18
delirium tremens 301
dementia
 corticobasal degeneration 108
 fronto-temporal 98
 fronto-temporal with parkinsonism 117
 with Lewy bodies 36
 myoclonus 191
 Parkinson's disease 36, 68
 pugilistica 121
dentatorubropallidoluysian atrophy (DRPLA) 165, 187, 188, 282
depression 68
desmopressin 104
diabetes 333
diffusion-weighted imaging 40
distractibility 318, 320, 322, 324
*DJ-1* 43
*DNAJC6* 44
doll's head manoeuvre 97
donepezil 68
dopa-responsive dystonia 210–11
dopamine
 basal ganglia circuits 14, 16, 20
 beta oscillations 18
dopamine agonist withdrawal syndrome 266
dopamine
 agonists 56–9, 67
dopamine dysregulation syndrome 80, 300
dopamine receptor blockers 152, 252, 254, 256
dopamine transporter deficiency syndrome 211
dorsolateral prefrontal loop 10
Down's syndrome 156
drooling 69
drug-induced disorders 249–66
 akathisia 265
 akinetic crisis 264–5
 chorea 161, 173, 258
 clinical presentation 250
 dopamine agonist withdrawal syndrome 266

dystonia 230, 254, 256
myoclonus 262
neuroleptic malignant
  syndrome 264
neuroleptic malignant
  syndrome-like
  syndromes 264–5
parkinsonism 252, 253
parkinsonism–
  hyperpyrexia
  syndrome 264–5
serotonin syndrome 265
tics 262
tremor 130, 260
withdrawal emergent
  syndrome 266
Duodopa® 52, 54, 78, 84
dyskinesia 2
  beginning-and-end-
    of-dose 79
  belly dancer's 311
  biphasic 79
  end-of-dose 79
  management in
    Parkinson's
    disease 78–9
  off-period 79
  peak-dose 78, 79
  square-wave 78
  tardive 256
dysphagia 71
dystonia 2, 195–248
  acquired 198, 230
  acute dystonic reac-
    tions 230, 254, 255
  adult-onset isolated
    cranio-cervical
    208–9, 235
  adult-onset isolated
    limb 206, 234
  amino acidaemias 219
  ataxia 215, 219
  blepharospasm 209,
    235, 242
  botulinum toxin 238–42
  brain injury 230
  causalgia–dystonia 321
  causes 198
  cerebellar syndrome 281
  cervical 208, 235, 240
  classification 196–7
  combined 197, 198, 200,
    210–19, 235
  constraint-induced
    movement
    therapy 246
  deafness 215, 219
  deep brain
    stimulation 244
  definition 196
  degenerative 214–16
  dopa-responsive 210–11

dopamine trans-
  porter deficiency
  syndrome 211
drug-induced 230,
  254, 256
dystonia-plus
  syndromes 196, 210
DYT1 204
DYT6 205
examination 201
eye movement
  disorders 214, 218
fixed 321
focal 196
functional 197, 320–1
generalized 196
genetic (DYT)
  classification 202
hemidystonia 196, 230
heredo-degenerative
  196, 216, 235
history-taking 201
infection 230
isolated 197, 198, 200,
  204–9, 234
laryngeal 209, 235
medical treatment 236
mirror
  movements 201, 206
monoamine neu-
  rotransmitter
  disorders 211, 213
multifocal 196
myoclonus 182
neuronal brain iron
  accumulation
  syndromes 219, 224–7
Oppenheim's 204
oromandibular 208, 235
pallidotomy 244
parkinsonism 214, 218
paroxysmal 197
peripheral
  neuropathy 215, 219
physical therapy 246
post-traumatic 321
primary 196
primary torsion 204
prominent bulbar
  involvement 214, 219
retraining therapy 246
secondary 196
segmental 196
sleep disorders 293
status dystonicus 232
surgical treatment 244
tardive 230, 256
torticollis 208
treatment 234–46
tremor 132, 133
Wilson's disease 220–3
writing 201, 206

young-onset generalized
  204–5, 234
dystonia-plus
  syndromes 196, 210
dystonic clenched fist 109

# E

ear, dyskinetic
  movements 311
early infantile myoclonic
  encephalopathy 184
echolalia 142
echopraxia 142
Ehlers–Danlos syndrome
  (type 3) 321
*EIF4G1* 43
Ekbom's syndrome (restless
  legs) 293, 294–5, 296
electroencephalography
  181, 184, 324
electromyography 104,
  181, 318, 324, 333
encephalitis
  lethargica 121, 230
encephalopathy 184, 190
enkephalin 20
entacapone 62
entrainment 318, 324
epilepsia partialis
  continua 184
epilepsy
  autosomal dominant
    nocturnal frontal
    lobe 273
  frontal lobe 273
  myoclonus 184, 186–8
  startle 330
episodic ataxias 268,
  276, 277
*EPM1* 186
Epstein–Barr virus 121
erectile
  dysfunction 69, 105
ergot dopamine
  agonists 56
essential tremor 132, 133
exercise-induced
  dyskinesia 271, 272
eye movements
  corticobasal
    degeneration 109
  dystonia 214, 218
  Huntington's disease 164
  parkinsonism 25
  progressive supranuclear
    palsy 97
  stiff-person
    syndrome 333
'eye of the tiger'
  sign 225, 228
eyelid apraxia 96, 242

## F

*FA2H*-associated neurodegeneration 225–6
facial myokimia 311
facio-brachial dystonic seizures 310–11
Fahr's syndrome 116
falls 75, 97
familial cortical tremor with or without epilepsy 182
familial fatal insomnia 301
fatigue 326
FBXO7 44
festinant gait 22
fibrosis 56
fixed dystonia 321
FMR1 286
focal dystonia 196
focal myoclonus 190
focal tremor syndromes 136–7
fragile X-associated tremor/ataxia syndrome 286
fragile X syndrome 156, 286
freezing 22, 75
Friedreich's ataxia 283, 284
Froment's manoeuvre 22
frontal lobe epilepsy 273
frontal lobe seizures 300
fronto-temporal dementia 98
  with parkinsonism. 117
functional movement disorders 3, 313–28
  diagnostic criteria 317
  dystonia 197, 320–1
  epidemiology 316
  examination 316
  gait disturbances 317
  history-taking 316
  management 326–7
  myoclonus 324
  parkinsonism 322
  prognostication 327
  tremor 134, 318
  types of 316
fungal infection 121
*FUS* 117, 118

## G

GABA 20
gabapentin 139
gait
  functional movement disorders 317
  functional parkinsonism 322
  parkinsonism 22, 25
  Parkinson's disease 75
Gaucher's disease 44
*GBA* 44
generalized dystonia 196
genetic counselling 166–7
genetic testing 41, 44
genetics
  dopa-responsive dystonia 210
  dystonia 202
  Huntington's disease 166
  Parkinson's disease 26, 42–4
  progressive supranuclear palsy 96
  Tourette's syndrome 151
*GIGYF2* 43
Gilles de la Tourette syndrome 148, 150–4
globus pallidus externa 14
globus pallidus interna 14
glucose transporter (GLUT1) deficiency 272, 273, 288
GM1 gangliosidosis 218
GM2 gangliosidosis 219
*GNAL* 208
*GOSR2* 188
*GTPCH1* 210
Guillain–Mollaret triangle 137, 288

## H

Hallervorden–Spatz syndrome 224
hallucinations 68–9
HARP syndrome 171
'hatter's shakes' 130
Haw River syndrome 187
HD-like syndrome 165, 171
head bobbing 136
head trauma 121
hemiballismus 125, 134, 136
hemiballismus (hemiballism) 18, 160
hemidystonia 196, 230
hemifacial spasm 306–8
hemi-masticatory spasm 310
hereditary ataxia with vitamin E deficiency 284
hereditary geniospasm 137
hereditary quivering chin 137
hereditary sensorimotor neuropathy 130
heredo-degenerative movement disorders 3
  dystonia 196, 216, 235
  parkinsonism 94

hiccups 176
*HIT* 166
HIV 121
Hoehn and Yahr staging 90
Holmes tremor 134
'hot cross bun' sign 104, 106
*HTRA2* 43
'hung-up jerk' 330
*huntingtin* 166
Huntington's disease 164–8
hyperekplexia 330
hyperkinetic movement disorders 2, 18
hypersexuality 80
hyperthyroidism 130
hypnogogic jerks 176
hypnopompic jerks 176
hypobetalipoproteinaemia 171
hypokinetic movement disorders 2, 18

## I

idiopathic basal ganglia calcification 116
idiopathic chronic motor or vocal tic disorder 148
idiopathic hemifacial spasm 306
idiopathic movement disorders 3
idiopathic simple transient tics of childhood 148
imaging
  corticobasal degeneration 109
  fragile X syndrome 286
  manganism 121
  multisystem atrophy 104, 106
  neuronal brain iron accumulation syndromes 225–6, 228
  Parkinson's disease 40–1
  progressive supranuclear palsy 98, 100
  Tourette's syndrome 150
immunoglobulin M paraproteinaemia 130
impulse control disorders 56
infection
  chorea 161
  dystonia 230
  parkinsonism 121
  tics 156–7
insomnia 80, 293, 300
intention tremor 124
intermanual conflict 108

# INDEX

internal segment of the globus pallidus 14
isolated movement disorders 3

## J

*jactatio capitis nocturnis* 300
Japanese B encephalitis 121, 230
jaw tremor 125, 136
*JPH3* 165, 171
jumping Frenchmen of Maine 330
juvenile myoclonic epilepsy 184

## K

Karak syndrome 225
Kayser–Fleischer rings 220, 221
*KCNA1* 276
kinetic tremor 124, 125, 134
Kufor–Rakeb syndrome 44, 117, 226
Kufs disease 186

## L

Lafora body disease 186, 188
Lance–Adams syndrome 190
laryngeal dystonia 209, 235
lateral orbito-frontal loop 10
'lead pipe' rigidity 22
Lee Silverman Voice Treatment 70
Lennox–Gastaut syndrome 184
lentiform nucleus 10
Lesch–Nyhan syndrome 156
lesion operations 7, 153, 244
levator inhibition 96, 242
levetiracetam 192
levodopa 52–4, 67, 211
levodopa challenge 40, 41
Lewy bodies 28
lightning jerks 182
*LINGO1* 132
liver biopsy 221
liver flap 169
long-term levodopa syndrome 53
*LRRK2* 42, 44
Lubag syndrome 218

## M

McLeod's syndrome 170–1
magnetic resonance imaging (MRI)
 fragile X syndrome 286
 manganism 121
 multisystem atrophy 104, 106
 neuronal brain iron accumulation syndromes 225–6,228
 Parkinson's disease 40
 progressive supranuclear palsy 98, 100
 Tourette's syndrome 150
manganese 120–1
mannerisms 142
*MAPT* 96
MDS Unified Parkinson's Disease Rating Scale 90
*MECP2* 156
medical treatment 6
Meige syndrome 208
melanoma 53
mental retardation 156
mercury 130
metabolic disturbances 130, 161
metachromatic leukodystrophy 219
methylphenidate 153, 262
MIBG scintigraphy 98, 104
'Mickey Mouse' sign 100
midbrain tremor 134
mild cognitive impairment 36
MIRAS 284
mirror movements 201, 206
mitochondrial membrane protein-associated neurodegeneration 225
mixed movement disorders 2
Mohr–Tranebjaerg syndrome 219
monoamine neurotransmitter disorders 211, 213
monoamine oxidase inhibitors 60, 67
monoballism 160
Morvan's syndrome 301
motor loop 10
motor recklessness 97
motor tics 142, 143
movement disorders
 basal ganglia circuits 18
 differential diagnosis 3
 hypokinetic versus hyperkinetic 2, 18
 investigation 4

management approaches 6–7
MPTP 121
*MR1* 271
MRI, see magnetic resonance imaging
multidisciplinary teams 48
multifocal dystonia 196
multisystem atrophy 102–5, 112, 218
myoclonic epilepsy with ragged red fibres 187, 188
myoclonus 2, 175–94
 acquired 177, 190–1
 Baltic 186
 benign neonatal sleep 300
 causes 176, 177
 cerebellar syndrome 281
 coeliac disease 191
 cortical 176
 definition and description 176
 dementia 191
 differential diagnosis 176
 drug-induced 262
 dystonia 182
 encephalopathy 184, 190
 epilepsy 184, 186–8
 examination 180
 familial cortical tremor with or without epilepsy 182
 focal 190
 functional 324
 history-taking 180
 inherited syndromes 177, 182, 184, 186–8
 investigation 180, 181
 negative 176
 neurodegeneration 177, 191
 opsoclonus–myoclonus 191
 paraneoplastic syndromes 191
 parkinsonism 191
 post-hypoxic 190
 progressive myoclonic epilepsy–ataxia syndromes 186–8
 propriospinal 190
 reticular reflex 190
 segmental 190
 sleep disorders 293, 300
 spinal segmental 190
 subacute sclerosing panencephalitis 191
 subcortical 176
 treatment 180, 192–3
myokimia 276, 311

## N

narcolepsy–cataplexy 301
neck–tongue syndrome 311
neural oscillations 18
neuroacanthocytosis 170, 219
neurodegeneration
 mechanism 114–15
 myoclonus 177, 191
 REM-sleep behaviour disorder 298
 tics 156
neuroferritinopathy 165, 227
neuroleptic malignant syndrome 264
neuroleptic malignant syndrome-like syndromes 264–5
neuromyotonia 276
neuronal brain iron accumulation syndromes 219, 224–7
neuronal ceroid lipofuscinoses 186, 188
neuronal intermediate filament inclusion disease 118
neuronal intranuclear inclusion disease 118
neuropathic tremor 130
neuroprotection 66
neuropsychiatric
 symptoms 38
 side effects of therapy 80
neurotransmitters
 in basal ganglia 20
 monoamine neurotransmitter disorders 211, 213
NICE guidance 49
Niemann–Pick type C 218
NMDA-antibody encephalitis 173, 301
non-obscene socially inappropriate behaviours 151
North Sea progressive myoclonus epilepsy 188
nurse specialists 88

## O

occupational therapy 70
oculo-masticatory myorhythmia 137, 310
oculomotor loop 10
Ohtahara syndrome 184
olanzapine 69
olfactory dysfunction 41

Oppenheim's dystonia 204
opsoclonus–myoclonus 191
oromandibular dystonia 208, 235
orthostatic hypotension 104
orthostatic tremor 136
OT-plus 136
Othello syndrome 56
oxybutinin 69, 104

## P

pain 326
painful arms and moving fingers 310
painful legs and moving toes 310
palatal tremor 125, 137
palilalia 142
pallidal degeneration syndromes 117
pallidotomy 244
PANDAS 156–7
pantothenate kinase-associated neurodegeneration 224–5
paraneoplastic stiff-person syndrome 334
paraneoplastic syndromes 191
PARK1–20 42–4
parkin 43
parkinsonism 2
 causes 22, 23, 94
 cerebellar syndrome 281
 degenerative causes 116–18
 description of 22
 drug-induced 252, 253
 dystonia 214, 218
 examination 24, 25
 functional 322
 heredo-degenerative 94
 history-taking 24
 infectious and post-infectious 121
 myoclonus 191
 secondary 23, 94, 120–1
 tardive 252
 toxins 120–1
 vascular 120
 see also atypical parkinsonism
parkinsonism–hyperpyrexia syndrome 264–5
Parkinson's disease 21–92
 amantadine 64
 anticholinergics 64, 67
 apathy 68

apomorphine 59, 82–3
autonomic symptoms 38, 69
autosomal dominant 42–4
autosomal recessive 43–4
basal ganglia circuits 18, 28
benign tremulous 128
breaking the news 46
catechol-O-methyltransferase inhibitors 62
clinical diagnosis 34, 35
continuous dopaminergic stimulation 78
deconditioning 66
deep brain stimulation 86–7
dementia 36, 68
depression 68
differentiating from atypical parkinsonism 112
dopamine agonists 56–9, 67
drooling 69
Duodopa® 52, 54, 78, 84
dyskinesia management 78–9
dysphagia 71
dystonia 218
epidemiology 26
erectile dysfunction 69
escalation of treatment 74–6
examination 32
falls 75
fluctuations in symptom control 75
follow-up 72
freezing 75
gait disturbance 75
genetic risk 26
genetic testing 41, 44
genetics of 42–4
hallucinations 68–9
historical aspects 26
history-taking 30
Hoehn and Yahr staging 90
imaging 40–1
initiation of treatment 66–7
investigations 40–1
levodopa 52–4, 67
levodopa challenge 40, 41
management 48
MDS Unified Parkinson's Disease Rating Scale 90

## INDEX

measuring disease severity 90
mild cognitive impairment 36
monoamine oxidase inhibitors 60, 67
multidisciplinary teams 48
neuroprotection 66
neuropsychiatric side effects of therapy 80
neuropsychiatric symptoms 38
NICE guidance 49
non-motor symptoms 36, 38, 68–9
nurse specialists 88
occupational therapy 70
olfactory dysfunction 41
pathology 28
physiotherapy 70
prion-like disease 115
psychosis 68–9
sensory symptoms 38
sleep disturbances 38, 69, 80
speech and language therapy 70–1
titration of treatment 67
treatment of motor symptoms 50–67
treatment of non-motor symptoms 68–9
tremor 32, 128, 129
tremor-dominant 128
urinary dysfunction 69
Parkinson's disease–amyotrophic lateral sclerosis complex of Guam 117
paroxysmal dyskinesia 268, 270–4
paroxysmal dystonia 197
paroxysmal exercise-induced dyskinesia 271, 272
paroxysmal kinesigenic dyskinesia 270, 271
paroxysmal movement disorders 267–76
classification 268
dyskinesia 268, 270–4
episodic ataxias 268, 276, 277
pathophysiology 268
primary 268
secondary 268
treatment 268
paroxysmal nocturnal dyskinesia 273
paroxysmal non-kinesigenic dyskinesia 271

pathological gambling 80
patient expectations 4
penicillamine 222, 223
penicillamine challenge 221
pergolide 56, 59
periodic limb movements of sleep 293, 295, 296
peripheral neuropathy 130, 215, 219
Perry syndrome 117
PET 41, 104, 109
PGRN 117
phenylalanine loading test 210
phenytoin 274
phospholipase 2, group IV-associated neurodegeneration 225
physical therapy 246
physiological tremor 130
physiotherapy 70, 326
pill-rolling 22, 32, 128
pimozide 152, 154
PINK1 43
piracetam 192
piribedil 59
Pisa syndrome 102
PLA2G6 44, 225
polyarteritis nodosa 173
positron emission tomography (PET) 41, 104, 109
post-encephalitic parkinsonism 121
post-hypoxic myoclonus 190
post-infectious parkinsonism 121
post-traumatic dystonia 321
postural disturbances 22
postural tremor 124, 125, 129, 130–3
pramipexole 58, 59, 296
pregnancy 172
primary CNS vasculitis 173
primary dystonia 196
primary movement disorders 3
primary paroxysmal movement disorders 268
primary tics 142, 145, 148
primary torsion dystonia 204
primidone 139, 192
prion disease 115
progressive ataxia palatal tremor syndrome 137, 288
progressive cervical dystonia and ataxia 219

progressive encephalomyelitis with rigidity and myoclonus 334
progressive myoclonic epilepsy–ataxia syndromes 186–8
progressive non-fluent aphasia 98
progressive supranuclear palsy 96–9, 112, 218
propranolol 139
propriospinal myoclonus 190
PRRT2 270, 271
pseudo-athetosis 130
PSP-parkinsonism 98
psychiatric assessment 326
psychogenic movement disorders 3; *see also* functional movement disorders
psychological assessment 326
psychosis 68–9
pterins 210–11, 212
punding 80
pure akinesia with gait freezing 98
putamen 14

## R

RAB7L1 43
Ramsay–Hunt syndrome 186
rapid-onset dystonia parkinsonism 218
rasagiline 60
red flags 30, 32, 102, 157, 200
re-emergent tremor 32, 129
Refsum's disease 284
REM-sleep behaviour disorder 293, 298–301
rest tremor 22, 124, 125, 128–9
restless legs syndrome 293, 294–5, 296
reticular reflex myoclonus 190
retraining therapy 246
Rett's syndrome 156
Richardson's syndrome 98
rigidity 22, 322
risperidone 69, 152
rivastigmine 68, 69
ropinirole 58, 59, 296
rotigotine 58–9, 59, 296
rubral tremor 134

## S

saccades, see eye movements
Sandhoff disease 219
SANDO 284
scans without evidence of dopaminergic deficit (SWEDDs) 129
secondary dystonia 196
secondary movement disorders 3
secondary parkinsonism 23, 94, 120–1
secondary paroxysmal movement disorders 268
secondary tics 142, 145, 156–7
Segawa syndrome 210
segmental dystonia 196
segmental myoclonus 190
seizures
 facio-brachial dystonic 310–11
 sleep movement disorders 300
 see also epilepsy
selective serotonin reuptake inhibitors (SSRIs) 68
selegiline 60
SENDA 226
senile chorea 173
sensory symptoms 38
sepiapterin reductase deficiency 211
serotonergic crisis 60, 61
serotonin syndrome 265
sialidosis 187, 188
sildenafil 69, 105
simple tics 142, 143
single-photon emission computerized tomography 40, 109
*SLC2A1* 272
*SLC6A3* 211
sleep and sleep disturbances 291–302
 daytime somnolence 80, 293, 300
 disruption of normal sleep patterns 300
 dystonia 293
 insomnia 80, 293, 300
 myoclonus 293, 300
 narcolepsy–cataplexy 301
 NMDA-antibody encephalitis 301
 Parkinson's disease 38, 69, 80,
 paroxysmal nocturnal dyskinesia 273
 periodic limb movements of sleep 293, 295, 296
 REM-sleep behaviour disorder 293, 298–301
 restless legs syndrome 293, 294–5, 296
 seizures 300
 sleep attacks 56, 300
 status dissociatus 301
smoking 26
*SNCA* 44
sodium valproate 192
solvents 130
somatosensory evoked potentials 181
spasmodic torticollis 208
spasmus nutans 136
SPECT 40, 109
speech and language therapy 70–1
sphincter electromyography 104
spinal segmental myoclonus 190
spinocerebellar ataxia 219, 282
SSRIs 68
Stalevo® 52, 54, 62
startle epilepsy 330
startle syndromes 330
status dissociatus 301
status dystonicus 232
Steele–Richardson–Olszewski syndrome 96
stereotypies 142
stiff-limb syndrome 334
stiff-person syndrome 332–3
 paraneoplastic 334
streptococcal infection 121
striatum 14
subacute sclerosing panencephalitis 191
substance P 20
substantia nigra 15, 28
subthalamic nucleus 15
sulpiride 153–4
sunflower cataract 220
supportive treatment 6
surgical treatment 7
 dystonia 244
 hemifacial spasm 308
 Parkinson's disease 86–7
 Tourette's syndrome 153
 tremor 138
Sydenham's chorea 156, 172
syndromic associations 4
*SYNJ1* 44
synkinesis 22

## T

tardive dyskinesia 256
tardive dystonia 230, 256
tardive parkinsonism 252
tardive tic syndrome 262
tardive tremor 260
tau 96, 114
tauopathies 96, 108, 114
Tay–Sachs disease 219
tea-cup epilepsy 184
terminal tremor 124
tetrabenazine 152, 153, 236, 257
tetrathiomolybdate 222
*THAP1* 205
thumb, flexion tremor 128
thyroid–brain–lung syndrome 173
tic-tac jerks 182
tics 2, 141–58
 adult-onset tourettism 148
 brain injury 156
 classification 142
 complex 142, 143
 differential diagnosis 144
 drug-induced 262
 examination 145
 Gilles de la Tourette syndrome 148, 150–4
 history-taking 144
 idiopathic chronic motor or vocal tic disorder 148
 idiopathic simple transient tics of childhood 148
 infection 156–7
 investigation 145
 mental retardation 156
 motor 142, 143
 neurodegeneration 156
 primary 142, 145, 148
 secondary 142, 145, 156–7
 simple 142, 143
 suppression 142, 145
 tardive tic syndrome 262
 vocal 142, 143
tightrope walker gait 317
*TIMM8A* 219
*TITF-1* 173
titubation (head tremor) 125, 134, 136
tolcapone 62
tolterodine 69
topiramate 139
*TOR1A* 204
torticollis 208

Tourette's
 syndrome 148, 150–4
toxins
 parkinsonism 120–1
 tremor 130
transcranial sonography 41
tremor 2, 123–40
 action 124
 amplitude 124
 botulinum toxin 138
 causes 124, 125
 cerebellar 134
 cerebellar syndrome 281
 chin 125, 137
 deep brain
  stimulation 138
 definition 124
 describing 124
 drug-induced 130, 260
 dystonic 132, 133
 essential 132, 133
 examination 126–7
 focal tremor
  syndromes 136–7
 frequency 124
 functional 134, 318
 head 125, 134, 136
 history-taking 126
 Holmes 134
 intention 124
 investigation 127
 jaw 125, 136
 kinetic 124, 125, 134
 medical treatment 138–9
 metabolic
  disturbances 130
 midbrain 134
 mimics of 135
 neuropathic 130
 orthostatic 136
 palatal 125, 137
 parkinsonian 22
 Parkinson's disease 32,
  128, 129
 physiological 130
 postural 124, 125,
  129, 130–3
 re-emergent 32, 129
 rest 22, 124, 125, 128–9
 rubral 134
 surgical treatment 138
 tardive 260
 terminal 124
 toxins 130
 treatment 138–9
 wing-beating 134
 writing 132
trihexyphenidyl 64, 138,
 236, 257
trientene 222
trospium 69
*TUBB4A* 209
tuberculosis 121
tufted astrocytes 96
24-hour urinary
 copper 221
tyrosine hydroxylase
 deficiency 211

## U

*UCHL1* 42
UK Parkinson's Disease
 Society Brain
 BankClinical
 Criteria 34, 35
ultrasound 41
Unverricht–Lundborg
 disease 186, 188
urinary dysfunction 69, 104

## V

vascular parkinsonism 120
vocal tics 142, 143
voltage-gated potas-
 sium channel
 antibodies 301, 311
*VPS13A* 170
*VPS35* 43

## W

walking on ice gait 317
*WDR45* 226
websites
 ataxia 290
 atypical parkinsonism 122
 chorea 174
 dystonia 248
 functional movement
  disorders 328
 myoclonus 194
 Parkinson's disease 92
 sleep disturbances 302
 tics 158
 tremor 140
West Nile virus 121
West's syndrome 184
Whipple's disease 137
whispering dysphonia 209
Wilson's disease 220–3
wing-beating tremor 134
withdrawal emergent
 syndrome 266
Woodhouse–Sakati
 syndrome 219
writer's cramp 206
writing 132, 201, 206

## X

X-linked
 dystonia–deafness 219
X-linked dystonia
 parkinsonism 218
*XK* 170

## Y

young-onset generalized
 dystonia 204–5, 234

## Z

zinc 222, 223